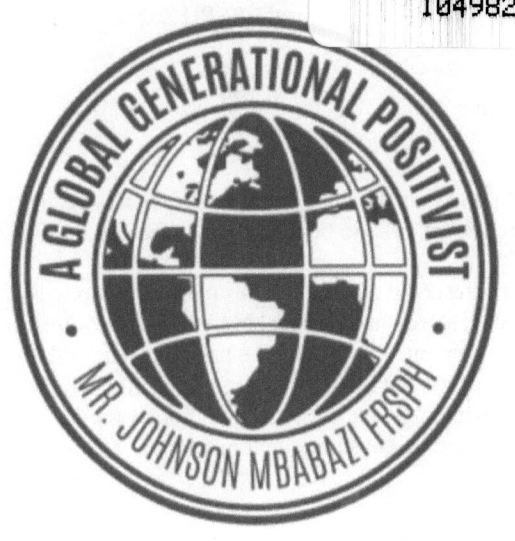

**Leukaemia
Mr. Johnson Mbabazi FRSPH**

**C:\Users\CC
LEEDS\Downloads\llll.jpg**

Published by New Generation Publishing in 2021

Copyright © Johnson Mbabazi FRSPH 2021

First Edition

The author asserts the moral right under the Copyright, Designs and Patents Act 1988 to be identified as the author of this work.

All Rights reserved. No part of this publication may be reproduced, stored in a retrieval system or transmitted, in any form or by any means without the prior consent of the author, nor be otherwise circulated in any form of binding or cover other than that which it is published and without a similar condition being imposed on the subsequent purchaser.

ISBN 978-1-80031-246-3

www.newgeneration-publishing.com

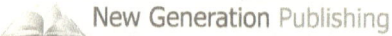

Contents

Abstract 1
Chapter 1 3
Introduction 3
Chronic lymphocytic leukaemia 4
Symptoms of CLL 4
Treatments for CLL 5
Outlook for CLL 6
Causes of CLL 6
Diagnosing chronic lymphocytic leukaemia 7
Some of the tests you might have are outlined below. 7
Blood tests 7
X-rays and scans 8
Bone marrow biopsy 8
Lymph node biopsy 9
Genetic tests 9
Treating chronic lymphocytic leukaemia 10
Stages of CLL 10
Monitoring early-stage CLL 11
Chemotherapy for more advanced CLL 11
Side effects of treatment 12
Stem cell or bone marrow transplants 13
Other treatments for CLL 14
Deciding against treatment 15
Complications of chronic lymphocytic leukaemia 15
Infections 15
Richter's syndrome 16

Autoimmune haemolytic anaemia 17
Psychological effects 17
Causes of chronic lymphocytic leukaemia 17
Family history 18
Ethnicity 18
Other medical conditions 18
Radiation exposure 19
Sex and age 19
Chronic myeloid leukaemia 20
What happens in chronic leukaemia 20
Warning signs of chronic myeloid leukaemia 21
How common is chronic myeloid leukaemia? 21
Outlook 22
Symptoms of chronic myeloid leukaemia 22
Causes of chronic myeloid leukaemia 23
Philadelphia chromosome 24
Possible triggers for chronic leukaemia 24
Benzene 24
Occupational risks 25
Other risk factors 25
Diagnosing chronic myeloid leukaemia 26
Bone marrow biopsy 26
Further tests 27
Cytogenetic testing 27
Polymerase chain reaction (PCR) 27
Imaging tests 27
Treating early-stage chronic myeloid leukaemia 29
    Imatinib 29

Nilotinib 29
Treating advanced chronic myeloid leukaemia 31
Chemotherapy 31
Bone marrow and stem cell transplants 32
Complications of chronic myeloid leukaemia 33
Symptoms of infection include: 33
Acute myeloid leukaemia 35
Signs and symptoms of AML 36
Seeking medical advice 36
What causes AML? 37
Who's affected 37
How AML is treated 38
Symptoms of acute myeloid leukaemia 38
Symptoms of AML 39
When to seek medical advice 40
Causes of acute myeloid leukaemia 40
Increased risk 40
The main risk factors for AML 41
   Radiation exposure 41
   Benzene and smoking 41
   Previous cancer treatment 41
   Blood disorders 42
   Genetic disorders 42
   Other suggested triggers 42
Diagnosing acute myeloid leukaemia 42
Bone marrow biopsy 43
Further tests 43
Genetic testing 43

Scans 44
Lumbar puncture 44
Treating acute myeloid leukaemia 45
Your treatment plan 45
   Treatment for AML is often carried out in two stages: 45
   Induction 46
   Intensive chemotherapy 46
Side effects of intensive chemotherapy for AML are common. 47
Non-intensive chemotherapy 48
All Trans-Retinoic Acid (ATRA) 48
Consolidation 48
The consolidation phase of treatment lasts several months. 49
Other treatments 49
Radiotherapy 49
Bone marrow and stem cell transplants 50
Azacitidine 50
Clinical trials and newer unlicensed treatments .. 51
Complications of acute myeloid leukaemia 51
Weakened immune system 51
Symptoms of an infection can include: 53
Serious bleeding can occur: 53
Infertility 54
Acute lymphoblastic leukaemia (ALL) 54
What is acute lymphoblastic leukaemia (ALL) ... 55
How common is ALL? 55
What happens in ALL 55

Blood cells and ALL	56
Types of leukaemia	57
In acute leukaemia:	57
In chronic leukaemia:	57
How leukaemia can affect you	58
Symptoms	58
General weakness	58
Frequent infections	59
Swollen lymph nodes	59
Pain in your bones or joints	60
Feeling short of breath (breathlessness)	60
Feeling full in your tummy (abdomen)	60
Pale skin	61
When to see your doctor	61
Symptoms of T cell ALL	61
Getting diagnosed	61
Risks and causes	62
Risk factors for ALL include:	62
Other possible causes	62
Risk factors for ALL and explanation	63
Ionising radiation exposure	63
Exposure to benzene	64
Smoking	64
Genetic conditions	64
Past chemotherapy	65
Viruses	65
Exposure to infection in childhood	65
Electromagnetic fields	66

House painting exposure 66
Weakened immunity 66
Treatment 67
Treatment options 67
Your MDT might include: 67
The main treatments for ALL 68
Other treatment 69
Phases of treatment 69
Getting rid of ALL (remission induction) 69
Treatment to stop ALL coming back (consolidation or intensification therapy) 70
Treating ALL that comes back or resists treatment 70
Clinical trials 71
Getting rid of ALL (remission induction) 72
Aim of the induction phase 72
What treatment to expect 72
Steroids 72
Chemotherapy into the spine 73
What happens next 73
Treatment to stop ALL coming back (consolidation therapy) 74
Aim of consolidation therapy 74
This phase of treatment might take a few months. 74
What treatment to expect 74
What happens next 75
Keeping ALL away long term (maintenance therapy) 75
What to expect 75
What happens next 76

Clinical trials	76
Chemotherapy for ALL	76
Phases of treatment for ALL	77
Aim of the induction phase	77
What treatment to expect	77
Steroids	78
Chemotherapy into the spine	78
What happens next	78
Treatment to stop ALL coming back (consolidation)	79
Keeping ALL away, long term (maintenance)	80
How you have chemotherapy	80
Side effects	81
Clinical trials	81
When at home	81
Chemotherapy drugs	82
Amsacrine (Amsidine, m-AMSA)	82
How it works	82
How you have it	82
Drugs into your bloodstream	83
When you have it	83
Tests	83
Other medicines, food and drink	83
Pregnancy and contraception	84
Fertility	84
Breastfeeding	84
Treatment for other conditions	84
Immunisations	84
Asparaginase (Crisantaspase, Erwinase)	85

- What is Asparaginase?.. 85
  - How it works 86
  - How you have it 86
  - Into your bloodstream 86
  - Injection into a muscle 86
  - Tests 87
  - Side effects 87
  - Other medicines, foods and drink................................ 87
  - Pregnancy and contraception 87
  - Fertility 87
  - Breastfeeding... 88
  - Immunisations 88
- Glucose and asparaginase 89
- Cyclophosphamide 89
  - How it works 89
  - How you have it 89
  - Drugs into your bloodstream 89
  - Taking your tablets.. 90
  - When you have it... 90
  - Tests 90
  - Other medicines, foods and drink................................ 90
  - Alcohol... 91
  - Pregnancy and contraception 91
  - Loss of fertility 91
  - Breastfeeding... 91
  - Treatment for other conditions 92
  - Immunisations 92
- Cytarabine (Ara C, cytosine arabinoside)........................ 93

- How it works 93
- How you have it 93
- Drugs into your bloodstream 93
- Subcutaneous injection... 94
- When you have it 94
- Tests 94
- Other medicines, foods and drink 94
- Pregnancy and contraception 95
- Loss of fertility.. 95
- Breastfeeding... 95
- Treatment for other conditions...................................... 95
- Immunisations 95

Daunorubicin 96
- How daunorubicin works 96
- How you have daunorubicin 97
- Into your bloodstream 97
- Central lines 97

Daunorubicin 97
- Tests 97
- Side effects.. 98
- When to contact your team 98
- Possible side effects 98

Coping with side effects 99
- What else do I need to know? 99
- Other medicines, foods and drink 99
- Pregnancy and contraception 100
- Fertility.. 100
- Breastfeeding... 100

- Treatment for other conditions 100
- Immunisations 100
- Doxorubicin (Adriamycin) 101
  - How doxorubicin works 102
  - How you have doxorubicin 102
  - Drugs into your bloodstream 102
  - Central lines 102
  - When you have it 102
  - Tests 103
  - Other medicines, foods and drink 103
  - Pregnancy and contraception 103
  - Fertility 103
  - Breastfeeding 104
  - Treatment for other conditions 104
  - If you have had radiotherapy 104
  - Immunisations 104
- Etoposide (Eposin, Etopophos, Vepesid) 105
  - How it works 105
  - How you have it 106
  - Drugs into your bloodstream 106
  - Taking capsules 106
  - Tests 107
  - Other medicines, foods and drink 107
  - Pregnancy and contraception 107
  - Breastfeeding 107
  - Loss of fertility 107
  - You may be able to store sperm before starting treatment 108

- Treatment for other conditions 108
- Immunisations 108

Mercaptopurine (Xaluprine) 109
- How it works 109
- How you have it 109
- Taking mercaptopurine tablets 109
- Taking mercaptopurine liquid 110
- If you take too much mercaptopurine 110
- Taking your tablets or capsules 111
- When you have it 111
- Tests 111
- Side effects 111
- When to contact your team 111
- Common side effects 112
- Increased risk of getting an infection 112
- Bruising, bleeding gums or nosebleeds 112
- Occasional side effects 113
- Rare side effects 113
- Other medicines, foods and drink 113
- Pregnancy and contraception 114
- Fertility 114
- Breastfeeding 114
- Treatment for other conditions 114
- Lactose and mercaptopurine 114
- Immunisations 115

Mercaptopurine (Xaluprine) 115
- How it works 116
- How you have it 116

- Taking mercaptopurine tablets 116
- Taking mercaptopurine liquid 116
- If you take too much mercaptopurine 117
- If you forget to take mercaptopurine 117
- Taking your tablets or capsules 117
- When you have it 117
- Tests 118
- Side effects 118
- When to contact your team 118
- Common side effects 119
- Increased risk of getting an infection 119
- Occasional side effects 119
- Rare side effects 120
- What else do I need to know? 120
- Other medicines, foods and drink 120
- Pregnancy and contraception 120
- Fertility 120
- Breastfeeding 121
- Treatment for other conditions 121
- Lactose and mercaptopurine 121
- Immunisations 121

Methotrexate 122
- How methotrexate works 122
- How you have methotrexate 123
- Central lines 123
- Taking your tablets or liquid 123
- Injection into your muscle (intramuscular) 123
- When you have methotrexate 124

Tests	124
Side effects	125
When to contact your team	125
Common side effects	125
Increased risk of infection	125
Bruising, bleeding gums and nosebleeds	126
Mouth sores and ulcers	126
Liver changes	126
Indigestion or heartburn	126
Tummy (abdominal) pain	127
Feeling or being sick	127
Loss of appetite	127
Kidney changes	127
Occasional side effects	127
Rare side effects	128
Other medicines, foods and drink	129
Avoid drinking alcohol while having methotrexate	129
Pregnancy and contraception	129
Breastfeeding	129
Treatment for other conditions	130
Fertility	130
Driving and use of machinery	130
Immunisations	130
Methotrexate	131
How methotrexate works	131
How you have methotrexate	132
Central lines	132
When you have methotrexate	133

Tests 133
Side effects 134
When to contact your team 134
Common side effects 134
Increased risk of infection 134
Bruising, bleeding gums and nosebleeds 135
Mouth sores and ulcers 135
Liver changes 135
Indigestion or heartburn 135
Tummy (abdominal) pain 136
Feeling or being sick 136
Loss of appetite 136
Kidney changes 136
Occasional side effects 136
Rare side effects 137
Other medicines, foods and drink 138
Breastfeeding 138
Treatment for other conditions 138
Fertility 139
Driving and use of machinery 139
Immunisations 139

Nelarabine (Atriance) 140
How it works 140
Drugs into your bloodstream 141
Central lines 141
Tests 142
Other medicines, foods and drink 142
Sodium and nelarabine 143

- Pregnancy and contraception 143
- Fertility 143
- Breastfeeding 143
- Treatment for other conditions 143
- Immunisations 144

Tioguanine (thioguanine, 6-TG, 6-tioguanine) 144
- How it works 145
- How you have it 145
- Taking your tablets 145
- When you have tioguanine 146
- Tests 146
- Other medicines, foods and drink 146
- Pregnancy and contraception 146
- Fertility 146
- Breastfeeding 147
- Treatment for other conditions 147

Lesche-Nyhan syndrome 147
TPMT (thiopurine methyltransferase) 147
- Immunisations 148

Vincristine 148
- How it works 149
- How you have it 149
- Drugs into your bloodstream 149
- Tests 149
- Side effects 149
- When to contact your team 150
- Hair loss 151

Tiredness and weakness (fatigue) during and after treatment 151
Feeling or being sick 151
Constipation 151
Tummy (abdominal) pain 152
Muscle or bone pain 152
Sore mouth and throat 152
Swelling and pain at the drip site 153
Allergic reaction 153
Taste changes 153
Hearing changes 153
Loss of appetite and weight loss 153
Skin rash 154
Headaches 154
Diarrhoea 154
Other medicines, foods and drink 155
Pregnancy and contraception 155
Fertility 155
Breastfeeding 155
Treatment for other conditions 155
Immunisations 156
Steroids 156
How you have steroids 157
Having an injection into a muscle or a vein 157
Taking medications safely 157
Side effects 157
Changes to blood sugar levels 158
Targeted cancer drugs and immunotherapy 159

- Targeted cancer drugs 159
  - Side effects 160
- Drugs that help the body's immune system (immunotherapy) 160
  - Side effects 161
- CAR T-cell therapy 161
- Types of targeted cancer drugs and immunotherapy for ALL 162
- Imatinib (Glivec) 162
  - How it works 162
  - How you have it 163
  - Taking your tablets 163
  - When you have it 163
  - Tests 163
  - Side effects 164
  - When to contact your team 164
  - Common side effects 165
  - Increased risk of getting an infection 165
  - Breathlessness and looking pale 165
  - Bruising, bleeding gums or nosebleeds 165
  - Tiredness and weakness (fatigue) 165
  - Fluid build-up (oedema) 166
  - Feeling or being sick 166
  - Diarrhoea 166
  - Headaches 166
  - Indigestion 166
  - Skin rash 167
  - Muscle and joint pain 167

- Weight gain 167
- Tummy (abdominal) pain 167
- Occasional side effects 167
- Rare side effects 168
- Other medicines, foods and drink................................. 168
- Pregnancy and contraception 169
- Fertility 169
- Breastfeeding... 169
- Treatment for other conditions..................................... 169
- Immunisations 169
- Children and adolescents.. 170

Dasatinib (Sprycel) 171
How it works 171
How you have it... 171
- Taking your tablets 172
- Tests 172
- Side effects 172
- When to contact your team 173
- Common side effects 173
- Increased risk of getting an infection 173
- Berathlessness and looking pale................................... 173
- Bruising, bleeding gums or nosebleeds....................... 174
- Diarrhoea 174
- Headaches 174
- Skin changes.. 174
- Fluid build-up (oedema).. 175
- Feeling or being sick 175
- Bone or muscle pain.. 175

- Occasional side effects 175
- Rare side effects 176
- Coping with side effects 177
- Other medicines, foods and drink 177
- Pregnancy and contraception 177
- Fertility 177
- Breastfeeding 178
- Treatment for other conditions 178
- Immunisations 178

Ponatinib (Iclusig) 179
- How it works 179
- How you have it 180
- Taking your tablets or capsules 180
- When you have it 180
- Tests 180
- Side effects 180
- When to contact your team 181

Common side effects 181
- Increased risk of getting an infection 181
- Breathless and looking pale 182
- Bruising, bleeding gums or nosebleeds 182
- Skin changes 182
- Pain 182
- Headaches 182
- Dizziness 182
- High blood pressure 183
- Cough 183
- Loss of appetite 183

- Difficulty sleeping 183
- Tiredness and weakness (fatigue) 183
- Feeling or being sick 184
- Fluid build-up (swelling) 184
- Constipation 184
- Diarrhoea 184
- Occasional side effects 184
- Rare side effects 185
- Possible long term side effects 186
- Other medicines, foods and drinks 186
- Pregnancy and contraception 186
- Breastfeeding 186
- Fertility 187
- Treatment for other conditions 187
- Immunisations 187

Radiotherapy 188
Planning radiotherapy 188
- Injection of dye 189
- Having the scan 189
- Radiotherapy treatment mask 189
- Before making the mask 190
- Making the mask 190
- Injection of dye 191
- Having the scan 191
- Radiotherapy treatment mask (shell) 191
- Before making the mask 192
- Making the mask 192

Radiotherapy planning for TBI 192

Total body irradiation	193
After your planning session	193
Radiotherapy to the brain	193
Before treatment	194
The radiotherapy room	194
Before each treatment	194
During the treatment	195
Side effects	195
Possible long term side effects	196
Total body radiotherapy (TBI)	196
The radiotherapy room	196
Before treatment	197
During treatment	197
After treatment	198
Side effects	198
Possible long term effects	199
Growth factors	199
When you have growth factors	199
After chemotherapy	199
Before stem cell collection for a transplant	200
How you have growth factors	200
Growth factor type	200
Side effects	201
Stem cell or bone marrow transplants	201
What is a stem cell or bone marrow transplant?	201
What are stem cells?	201
How transplants work	202
A stem cell or bone marrow transplant	203

Why you might have a transplant 204
Types of transplant 204
Finding a donor.. 205
Stages of a donor stem cell transplant 205
Stages of a donor stem cell transplant 206
Donor's stem cell collection or harvest 206
Blood count recovery... 207
Collecting stem cells.. 207
Collecting your donor's stem cells from the blood 207
Preparing for the stem cell collection 208
On collection day... 208
Side effects of a stem cell collection 208
What happens 209
Recovery.. 209
Side effects of a transplant... 210
Side effects of high dose chemotherapy 210
Side effects of radiotherapy... 211
Fertility 212
Graft versus host disease 212
GvHD can be acute or chronic....................................... 213
Side effects of treatment.. 213
What side effects are.. 214
Side effects might be immediate or long term............... 215
Immediate side effects 215
Late effects 215
Coping with late effects... 216
Long terms side effects of treatment 216
Possible side effects... 217

Children may have puberty later than normal. 218
Coping with late effects 218

Abstract

Leukaemia is a type of blood cancer, which starts in blood-forming tissue, such as the bone marrow, and causes large numbers of immature blood cells to be produced and enter the bloodstream. Leukaemia is subdivided into different subtypes according to cellular maturity (acute or chronic) and cell type (lymphocytic or myeloid). The mainstays of leukaemia treatment for adults have been chemotherapy, radiation therapy, and stem cell transplantation. There different types of leukaemia that require different combinations of therapies. Although much progress has been made against some types of leukaemia, others still have relatively poor rates of survival. And, as the population ages, there is a greater need for treatment regimens that are less toxic. Acute Lymphoblastic Leukaemia (ALL) Combining less-toxic therapies. The intensive chemotherapy treatments used for ALL have serious side effects that many older patients cannot tolerate. Targeted therapies may have fewer side effects than chemotherapy. Researchers are developing clinical trials that will test whether combinations of these types of therapies can be used instead of chemotherapy for older patients with a form of ALL called B-cell ALL. Using CAR T-cell therapy. CAR T-cell therapy is a type of treatment in which a patient's own immune cells are genetically modified to treat their cancer. Currently, CAR T cells are approved for the treatment of some children and young adults with ALL. They are now being explored for use in older adults with B-cell ALL. Scientists hope that it will be possible to use CAR

T-cell therapy to delay or even replace stem-cell transplantation in older, frailer patients. A major challenge in treating another type of ALL, called T-cell ALL, has been that it can be resistant to chemotherapy and radiation therapy. Researchers are working to develop clinical trials to test new drugs that could potentially help counter this resistance. Acute Myeloid Leukaemia (AML); Targeted therapy. AML tends to be aggressive and is harder to treat than ALL. However, AML cells may have gene changes that can be targeted with new drugs. Targeted therapies that have recently been approved for AML include: Enasidenib (Idhifa), Venetoclax (Venclexta), Midostaurin (Rydapt) and Gilteritinib (Xospata). Researchers are also testing other ways to treat AML such as Looking at newer targeted therapies. One promising drug, called pevonedistat, targets a protein called NAE that is involved in cell division and is being studied in clinical trials.

Chapter 1

Introduction

Leukaemia is cancer of the white blood cells. Acute leukaemia means the condition progresses rapidly and aggressively and requires immediate treatment.

C:\Users\CC LEEDS\Downloads\llll.jpg

Acute leukaemia is classified according to the type of white blood cells affected by cancer. There are two main types:

- lymphocytes, which are mostly used to fight viral infections
- neutrophils, which perform several functions, such as fighting bacterial infections, defending the body against parasites and preventing the spread of tissue damage

Let me first focus on acute lymphoblastic leukaemia, which is cancer of the lymphocytes. The following other types of leukaemia are covered elsewhere:

- chronic lymphocytic leukaemia
- chronic myeloid leukaemia
- acute myeloid leukaemia

Chronic lymphocytic leukaemia

Chronic lymphocytic leukaemia is a type of cancer that affects the white blood cells and tends to progress slowly over many years.

It mostly affects people over the age of 60 and is rare in people under 40. Children are almost never affected.

In chronic lymphocytic leukaemia (CLL), the spongy material found inside some bones (bone marrow) produces too many white blood cells called lymphocytes that aren't fully developed and don't work properly.

Over time this can cause a range of problems, such as an increased risk of picking up infections, persistent tiredness, swollen glands in the neck, armpits or groin, and unusual bleeding or bruising.

CLL is different from other types of leukaemia, including chronic myeloid leukaemia, acute lymphoblastic leukaemia and acute myeloid leukaemia.

Symptoms of CLL

CLL doesn't usually cause any symptoms early on and may only be picked up during a blood test carried out for another reason.

When symptoms develop, they may include:

- getting infections often
- anaemia – persistent tiredness, shortness of breath and pale skin

- bleeding and bruising more easily than normal
- a high temperature (fever)
- night sweats
- swollen glands in your neck, armpits or groin
- swelling and discomfort in your tummy
- unintentional weight loss

You should visit doctor if you have any persistent or worrying symptoms. These symptoms can have other causes other than cancer, but it's a good idea to get them checked out.

Treatments for CLL

- As CLL progresses slowly and often has no symptoms at first, you may not need to be treated immediately.
- If it's caught early on, you will have regular check-ups over the following months or years to see if it's getting any worse.
- If CLL starts to cause symptoms, or isn't diagnosed until later on, the main treatments are:
- chemotherapy – where medication is taken as a tablet or given directly into a vein is used to destroy the cancerous cells.
- a stem cell or bone marrow transplant – where donated cells called stem cells are transplanted into your body so you start to produce healthy white blood cells.

Treatment can't usually cure CLL completely, but can slow

its progression and lead to periods where there are no symptoms. Treatment may be repeated if the condition comes back.

Outlook for CLL

- The outlook for CLL depends on how advanced it is when it's diagnosed, how old you are when diagnosed, and your general health.
- Younger, healthier people who are diagnosed when CLL is still in the early stages generally have the best outlook.
- Although it can't normally be cured, treatment can help control the condition for many years.
- Overall, around three in every four people with CLL will live at least five years after diagnosis, but this can range from 10 years or more if caught early on, to less than a year if caught at a very advanced stage.

Causes of CLL

- It's not clear what causes CLL. There's no proven link with radiation or chemical exposure, diet or infections. You can't catch it from anyone else or pass it on.
- However, having certain genes can increase your chances of developing CLL. You may be at a slightly higher risk of it if you have a close family member with it, although this risk is still small.

Diagnosing chronic lymphocytic leukaemia

Most cases of chronic lymphocytic leukaemia (CLL) are detected during blood tests carried out for another reason.

However, you should visit your doctor if you have worrying symptoms of CLL, such as persistent tiredness, unusual bleeding or bruising, unexplained weight loss or night sweats.

Your doctor may:

- ask about your symptoms and your medical and family history
- carry out a physical examination to check for problems such as swollen glands and a swollen spleen
- send off a blood sample for testing

If your doctor thinks you could have CLL, you will be referred to a hospital doctor called a haematologist, a specialist in blood disorders, for further tests.

Some of the tests you might have are outlined below.

Blood tests

- The main test used to help diagnose CLL is a type of blood test called a full blood count.
- This is where the number and appearance of the different blood cells in a sample of your blood are checked

in a laboratory.

- An abnormally high number of unusual white blood cells (lymphocytes) can be a sign of CLL. A detailed examination of these cells can usually confirm the diagnosis.

X-rays and scans

You may also have:

- a chest X-ray
- an ultrasound scan of your tummy
- a computerised tomography (CT) scan

These tests can check for problems caused by CLL, such as swollen glands or a swollen spleen, and help rule out other possible causes of your symptoms.

Bone marrow biopsy

- Sometimes the haematologist may recommend removing a sample of your bone marrow (bone marrow biopsy) so they can examine it under a microscope to check it for cancerous cells.
- The sample is removed using a needle inserted into your hip bone. Local anaesthetic is normally used to numb the area where the needle is inserted, although you may experience some discomfort during the biopsy.
- The procedure will last around 15 minutes and you

shouldn't need to stay in hospital overnight. You may have some bruising and discomfort for a few days afterwards.

Lymph node biopsy

- In some cases, removing and examining a swollen lymph gland can help confirm a diagnosis of CLL. This is known as a lymph node biopsy.
- The gland is removed during a minor operation carried out under either local or general anaesthetic, where you're asleep. You won't usually need to stay in hospital overnight.
- After the operation, you'll be left with a small wound that will be closed with stitches.

Genetic tests

- Tests may also be carried out on your blood and bone marrow samples to check for any unusual genes in the cancerous cells.
- Identifying unusual genes in these cells can help your doctors decide how soon you should start treatment and which treatment is best for you.
- Some treatments for CLL don't work as well in people with certain abnormal genes in the affected cells.

Treating chronic lymphocytic leukaemia

- Treatment for chronic lymphocytic leukaemia (CLL) largely depends on what stage the condition is at when it's diagnosed.
- You may just need to be monitored at first if it's caught early on. Chemotherapy is the main treatment if it's more advanced.
- Treatment can often help keep CLL under control for many years.
- It may go away after treatment initially (known as remission), but will usually come back (relapse) a few months or years later and may need to be treated again.

Stages of CLL

Doctors use "stages" to describe how far CLL has developed and help them determine when it needs to be treated.

There are three main stages of CLL:

- stage A – you have enlarged lymph glands in fewer than three areas (such as your neck, armpit or groin) and a high white blood cell count
- stage B – you have enlarged lymph glands in three or more areas and a high white blood cell count
- stage C – you have enlarged lymph glands or an enlarged spleen, a high white blood cell count, and a low red blood cell or platelet count

Stage B and C CLL are usually treated straight away. Stage A generally only needs to be treated if it's getting worse quickly or starting to cause symptoms.

Monitoring early-stage CLL

Treatment may not be needed if you don't have any symptoms when you're diagnosed with CLL.

This is because:

- CLL often develops very slowly and may not cause symptoms for many years
- there's no benefit in starting treatment early
- treatment can cause significant side effects

In these cases, you will normally just need regular visits to your doctor and blood tests to monitor the condition.

Treatment with chemotherapy will usually only be recommended if you develop symptoms, or tests show that the condition is getting worse.

Chemotherapy for more advanced CLL

Many people with CLL will eventually need to have chemotherapy. This involves taking medication to keep the cancer under control. There are a number of different medicines for CLL, but most people will take three main medications in treatment cycles lasting 28 days.

These medicines are:

- fludarabine – usually taken as a tablet for three to five

days at the start of each treatment cycle
- cyclophosphamide – also usually taken as a tablet for three to five days at the start of each treatment cycle
- rituximab – given into a vein over the course of a few hours (intravenous infusion) at the start of each treatment cycle
- Fludarabine and cyclophosphamide can usually be taken at home. Rituximab is given in hospital, and sometimes you may need to stay in hospital overnight.

A number of different medicines can also be tried if you can't have these medicines, you've tried them but they didn't work, or your CLL has come back after treatment.

These include bendamustine, chlorambucil, ibrutinib, idelalisib, obinutuzumab, ofatumumab and prednisolone (a steroid medication).

Side effects of treatment

The medicines used to treat CLL can cause some significant side effects, including:
- persistent tiredness
- feeling sick
- an increased risk of infections
- easy bruising or bleeding
- anaemia – shortness of breath, weakness and pale skin
- hair loss or thinning

- an irregular heartbeat
- an allergic reaction

Most side effects will pass once treatment stops. Let your care team know if you experience any side effects, as there are some treatments that can help.

Stem cell or bone marrow transplants

Stem cell or bone marrow transplants are sometimes used to try to get rid of CLL completely, or control it for longer periods.

Stem cells are cells produced by the spongy material found in the centre of some bones (bone marrow) that can turn into different types of blood cells, including white blood cells.

A stem cell transplant involves:

- having high-dose chemotherapy and radiotherapy to destroy the cancerous cells in your body
- removing stem cells from the blood or bone marrow of a donor – this will ideally be someone closely related to you, such as a sibling
- transplanting the donor stem cells directly into one of your veins

This is the only potential cure for CLL, but it's not done very often as it's an intensive treatment and many people with CLL are older and not well enough for the benefits to outweigh the risks. The initial treatment with chemotherapy and radiotherapy can place a significant strain on your body and cause troublesome side effects. There's also a risk of serious problems after the transplant, such as graft versus host disease. This is where the transplanted cells attack the other cells in your body.

Other treatments for CLL

There are also a number of other treatments that are sometimes used to help treat some of the problems caused by CLL, particularly if you can't have chemotherapy or it doesn't work.

These include:

- radiotherapy to shrink enlarged lymph glands or a swollen spleen
- surgery to remove a swollen spleen
- antibiotics, antifungals and antiviral medications to help reduce your risk of picking up an infection during treatment
- blood transfusions to provide more red blood cells and platelets (clotting cells) if you experience severe anaemia or problems with bleeding and bruising
- immunoglobulin replacement therapy – a transfusion of antibodies taken from donated blood that can help prevent infections
- injections of medication called granulocyte-colony stimulating factor (G-CSF) to help boost the number of white blood cells
- You may also need additional treatment for any complications of CLL that develop.

Deciding against treatment

As many of the treatments for CLL can have unpleasant side effects that may affect your quality of life, you may decide against having a particular type of treatment. This is entirely your decision and your treatment team will respect any decision you make. You won't be rushed into deciding about your treatment, and before making a decision you can talk to your doctor, partner, family and friends. Pain relief and nursing care will still be available as and when you need it.

Complications of chronic lymphocytic leukaemia

Chronic lymphocytic leukaemia (CLL) can sometimes cause a number of further complications. Some of the main problems people with the condition may experience are outlined below.

Infections

People with CLL usually have a weakened immune system and are more vulnerable to infections because they have a lack of healthy, infection-fighting white blood cells.

Treatment with chemotherapy can also further weaken the immune system.

If you have CLL, it's a good idea to:

☐ report any possible symptoms of an infection to your doctor or care team immediately – things to look out for include a high temperature (fever), aching muscles, diarrhoea or headaches

- ensure your vaccinations are up-to-date – speak to your doctor or care team for advice about any additional vaccines you might need, as some aren't safe if you have a weak immune system
- avoid close contact with anyone who has an infection – even if it's an infection to which you were previously immune, such as chickenpox

You may also be prescribed regular doses of medications such as antibiotics to help reduce the risk of infection.

Richter's syndrome

In up to 1 in every 20 people with CLL, the condition will change to become very similar to an aggressive form of non-Hodgkin lymphoma. This is called Richter's transformation or Richter's syndrome.

Symptoms of Richter's syndrome include:

- sudden swelling of your lymph glands
- a high temperature (fever)
- night sweats
- unintentional weight loss
- tummy (abdominal) pain

Richter syndrome is usually treated with a combination of chemotherapy and other powerful medicines.

Autoimmune haemolytic anaemia

Around 1 in every 10 people with CLL will develop a condition called autoimmune haemolytic anaemia. This is where the immune system starts to attack and destroy red blood cells. It can cause severe anaemia, making you feel breathless and easily tired. It's usually treated with steroid medication

Psychological effects

Being diagnosed with CLL can be very distressing and difficult to take in at first, particularly as it can't necessarily be cured and you may be advised to wait for it to get worse before starting treatment. Having to wait years to see how the condition develops can also be very stressful and make you feel anxious or depressed. Speak to your doctor or care team if you are finding it difficult to cope.

Causes of chronic lymphocytic leukaemia

It's not known what causes most cases of leukaemia. However, there are many risk factors that are known to increase your chances of getting chronic lymphocytic leukaemia.

Risk factors for chronic lymphocytic leukaemia include:

☐ having a family history of the condition

☐ being of European, American or Australian origin

☐ having certain medical conditions

☐ being male

These are discussed in more detail below.

Family history

In some cases, chronic lymphocytic leukaemia appears to run in families. It's thought that an inherited gene mutation (change to a gene) could increase your susceptibility to developing the condition. This means there may be certain genes in your family that make it more likely that you will develop chronic lymphocytic leukaemia. More research is needed, but having a parent or sibling (brother or sister) with chronic lymphocytic leukaemia slightly increases your chances of also developing the condition.

Ethnicity

Chronic lymphocytic leukaemia most commonly affects people of European, American and Australian origin. It's rare in people from China, Japan and South East Asia, and it affects more white people than black people. It's not known why the condition affects people of some ethnic backgrounds and not others.

Other medical conditions

Research has shown that having certain medical conditions slightly increases your chances of developing chronic lymphocytic leukaemia. These conditions include:

- pneumonia (chest infection)
- sinusitis
- shingles
- autoimmune haemolytic anaemia
- long-term (chronic) osteoarthritis
- prostatitis (an inflamed prostate)

However, rather than causing chronic lymphocytic leukaemia, some of these conditions may occur as a result of having lowered immunity during the early stages of the condition. Having a lowered immunity due to having a condition such as HIV or AIDS, or taking immunity lowering medication following an organ transplant can also increase your risk of developing chronic lymphocytic leukaemia.

Radiation exposure

Exposure to radiation is known to increase the risk of getting other types of leukaemia, but it's not been linked specifically to chronic lymphocytic leukaemia.

Sex and age

For reasons that are unclear, men are around twice as likely to develop chronic lymphocytic leukaemia than women. The risk of developing leukaemia also increases as you get older.

Chronic myeloid leukaemia

Leukaemia is cancer of the white blood cells. Chronic leukaemia means the condition progresses slowly over many years. Chronic leukaemia is classified according to the type of white blood cells that are affected by cancer. There are two main types:

- lymphocytes – mostly used to fight viral infections
- myeloid cells – which perform a number of different functions, such as fighting bacterial infections, defending the body against parasites and preventing the spread of tissue damage

These pages focus on chronic myeloid leukaemia, which is a cancer of the myeloid cells. The following other types of leukaemia are covered elsewhere:

- chronic lymphocytic leukaemia
- acute myeloid leukaemia
- acute lymphoblastic leukaemia

What happens in chronic leukaemia

Your bone marrow produces stem cells. These are unique cells because they have the ability to develop into three important types of blood cell:

- red blood cells – which carry oxygen around the body
- white blood cells – which help fight infection
- platelets – which help stop bleeding

In leukaemia, a genetic mutation in the stem cells causes a

huge over-production of white blood cells and a corresponding drop in red blood cells and platelets.

It's this lack of red blood cells which causes symptoms of anaemia, such as tiredness, and the lack of platelets that increases the risk of excessive bleeding.

Warning signs of chronic myeloid leukaemia

In its early stages, chronic myeloid leukaemia usually causes no noticeable symptoms. As the condition develops, symptoms include:

- tiredness
- weight loss
- night sweats
- a feeling of bloating
- bruising
- bone pain

How common is chronic myeloid leukaemia?

Chronic myeloid leukaemia is quite a rare type of cancer. Around 8,600 people are diagnosed with leukaemia every year in the UK. In 2011, around 680 people in the UK were diagnosed with chronic myeloid leukaemia. Chronic myeloid leukaemia can affect people of any age, but it is more common in people aged 40-60. There is no evidence that it runs in families.

Outlook

The outlook for chronic myeloid leukaemia depends to a large extent on how well a person responds to medication. Most patients (60-65%) do well on imatinib tablets, which are taken every day for life. For those who don't do well on imatinib, more than half respond to one of the alternative drugs. Nilotinib is recommended by the National Institute for Health and Care Excellence (NICE) for patients with chronic myeloid leukaemia who are not responding to, or can't tolerate imatinib. Those who fail these drugs or cannot tolerate them may be offered a bone marrow transplant if this is a suitable treatment. If the condition is diagnosed early (the chronic phase), the outlook is excellent, with almost 90% of people living at least five years after diagnosis.

Symptoms of chronic myeloid leukaemia

In its early stages, chronic myeloid leukaemia usually causes no noticeable symptoms and it is often diagnosed during tests for a different condition.

When symptoms do develop, they are similar to those of many other illnesses and can include:

- tiredness
- frequent infections
- unexplained weight loss

- a feeling of bloating
- less commonly, swollen lymph nodes – glands found in the neck and under your arms, which are usually painless

Chronic myeloid leukaemia can also cause swelling in your spleen (an organ that helps to filter impurities from your blood). This can cause a lump to appear on the left side of your abdomen, which may be painful when touched. A swollen spleen can also put pressure on your stomach, causing a lack of appetite and indigestion.

The symptoms of chronic myeloid leukaemia in its advanced stage will be much more noticeable and troublesome. They include:

- severe fatigue
- bone pain
- night sweats
- fever
- easily bruised skin

Causes of chronic myeloid leukaemia

Chronic myeloid leukaemia is caused by a DNA mutation in the stem cells which produce white blood cells. The change in the DNA causes the stem cells to produce more white blood cells than are needed. They are also released from the bone marrow before they are mature and able to fight infection like healthy 'adult' white blood cells. As the number of immature cells increases, the number of healthy red blood cells and platelets fall, and it's this fall which causes many of the symptoms of chronic leukaemia.

Philadelphia chromosome

Although the cause of chronic myeloid leukaemia is genetic, it is not inherited as it is an acquired genetic abnormality. Most people with the condition have an abnormal chromosome, where a section of DNA from one chromosome has been swapped with a section from another. This is called the Philadelphia chromosome and it makes the cell produce a protein that encourages the leukaemic cells to resist normal cell death and grow and multiply far more quickly than usual.

Possible triggers for chronic leukaemia

What triggers the development of chronic leukaemia and causes the initial mutation in stem cells is unknown. The one proven risk factor is exposure to radiation. However, radiation is only a significant risk if the levels are extremely high, such as those recorded after an atomic bomb explodes, or those released after a nuclear reactor accident, such as the one at Chernobyl.

Benzene

There is limited evidence that prolonged exposure to the chemical benzene leads to an increased risk of chronic myeloid leukaemia. Benzene is found in petrol and is also used in the rubber industry, but in the UK there are strict controls to protect people from prolonged exposure. Benzene is also found in cigarettes. However, it is thought that smoking is more of a risk factor in acute leukaemia than it is in chronic leukaemia.

Occupational risks

A number of occupations have been linked to an increased risk of chronic leukaemia, possibly due to exposure to certain substances such as pesticides or chemicals.

These occupations include:

- all types of agricultural workers
- people who are involved with rubber or plastic manufacture
- tailors and dressmakers
- cleaners
- builder's labourer

Other risk factors

There is some evidence to show an increased risk of chronic leukaemia in people who:

are obese

- have a weakened immune system – due to HIV or AIDS or taking immunosuppressant's after an organ transplant.
- have inflammatory bowel disease – such as ulcerative colitis or Crohn's disease

Diagnosing chronic myeloid leukaemia

Chronic myeloid leukaemia is often first detected when a routine blood test is carried out to diagnose another, unrelated, condition. A blood test that reveals abnormally high levels of white blood cells could be a sign of chronic leukaemia. If you have a blood test with abnormal results, you will be referred to a haematologist (a specialist in treating blood conditions) for further testing.

Bone marrow biopsy

To confirm a diagnosis of chronic leukaemia, the haematologist will take a small sample of your bone marrow to examine under a microscope. This procedure is known as a bone marrow biopsy. A bone marrow biopsy is usually carried out under a local anaesthetic. The haematologist will numb an area of skin at the back of your hip bone, before using a needle to remove the bone marrow sample. You may experience some pain once the anaesthetic wears off and some bruising and discomfort for a few days afterwards. The procedure takes around 15 minutes to complete and you should not have to stay in hospital overnight. The bone marrow sample will be checked to see if there are cancerous cells. If there are, the biopsy will also be able to help determine which type of chronic leukaemia is present.

Further tests

There are a number of additional tests that can be used to help reveal more information about the progress and extent of the leukaemia. These can also provide an insight into how the leukaemia should be treated. These are outlined below.

Cytogenetic testing

Cytogenetic testing involves identifying the genetic make-up of the cancerous cells. There are a number of specific genetic variations that can occur during leukaemia and knowing what these variations are can have an important impact on treatment. For example, 90% of people with chronic myeloid leukaemia have the Philadelphia chromosome. People who have this chromosome are known to respond well to a medicine called imatinib.

Polymerase chain reaction (PCR)

A polymerase chain reaction (PCR) test can be done on a blood sample. This is an important test to diagnose and monitor the response to treatment. The blood test is repeated every three months for at least two years after starting treatment, then less often once remission is achieved.

Imaging tests

In some cases, the hospital may want to perform some imaging tests to help rule out other conditions or confirm a diagnosis. This may be either:

- an X-ray – usually to examine your chest
- an ultrasound scan – usually to examine your spleen and liver

Treating chronic myeloid leukaemia

Imatinib tablets are usually given as soon as you have been diagnosed with chronic myeloid leukaemia, to slow its progression. These tablets are taken every day for life, and most patients do really well on them.

The aim of treatment is to achieve the following:

- by three months, correct the blood count
- by 12 months, clear the bone marrow of cells containing the Philadelphia chromosome (see Causes page for information on this)
- by 18 months, get to a stage where the leukaemia can only be detected by a very sensitive molecular test (molecular remission)
- Chemotherapy is usually offered if the cancer reaches an advanced stage.

These treatments are explained below.

Treating early-stage chronic myeloid leukaemia

Imatinib

A medicine called imatinib is the main treatment recommended for chronic myeloid leukaemia. It is usually given as soon as a diagnosis is made because the medicine is designed to slow the progression of the cancer and to prevent the condition reaching the accelerated or advanced phase. Imatinib is a type of tyrosine kinase inhibitor. This means it blocks a protein called tyrosine kinase (tyrosine kinase helps to stimulate the growth of cancer cells). This reduces the production of abnormal white blood cells.

Imatinib is taken as a tablet. The side effects of imatinib are usually mild and should improve with time. They include:

- nausea
- vomiting
- swelling in the face and lower legs
- muscle cramps
- rash
- diarrhoea

Nilotinib

It is estimated that 10-40% of people who take imatinib become resistant to its effects, so an alternative treatment is required. The National Institute for Health and Care Excellence (NICE) has recommended nilotinib for the treatment of chronic myeloid leukaemia that is resistant or intolerant to imatinib. In some cases, nilotinib is recommended as the first treatment. Nilotinib works in a similar way to imatinib in that it blocks the effects of proteins that help stimulate the growth of cancer cells.

Side effects of nilotinib can include:

- vomiting
- abdominal pain
- bone and joint pain
- dry skin
- loss of appetite
- hair loss
- insomnia
- night sweats
- dizziness
- tingling or numbness

If the side effects become particularly troublesome, temporarily stopping the treatment usually helps to bring them under control. Treatment can then be resumed, possibly using a lower dose of medication.

Treating advanced chronic myeloid leukaemia

Chemotherapy

Once chronic myeloid leukaemia has progressed to a more advanced stage, chemotherapy is the next treatment. Chemotherapy tablets are usually used first because they have fewer and milder side effects than chemotherapy injections. Side effects include:

- tiredness
- skin rash
- increased vulnerability to infection

Chemotherapy can weaken your immune system, which helps protect you against infection. This is known as being immunocompromised.

If your symptoms persist or get worse, chemotherapy injections (intravenous chemotherapy) will need to be used. Intravenous chemotherapy causes more side effects than chemotherapy tablets and they tend to be more severe.

Side effects include:

- nausea
- vomiting
- tiredness
- hair loss
- infertility

These side effects should resolve after your treatment has finished, although there is a risk that infertility could be permanent.

Bone marrow and stem cell transplants

A bone marrow transplant can offer a cure for chronic leukaemia, although it is only suitable and necessary for some patients. Before transplantation can take place, the person receiving the transplant has to have aggressive, high-dose chemotherapy and radiotherapy to destroy any cancerous cells in their body. This can put enormous strain on the body and can cause significant side effects and potential complications. Transplantations have better outcomes if the donor has the same tissue type as the person who is receiving the donation. The best candidate to provide a donation is usually a brother or sister with the same tissue type.

Due to these issues, transplantations are usually only successful when they are carried out in children and young people, or older people in good health, and there is a suitable brother or sister who can provide a donation. In most cases of chronic leukaemia, the potential risks of transplantation far outweigh any benefit. For example, the chances of an elderly person with advanced chronic leukaemia surviving a bone marrow transplant can be as low as one in five. However, your specific circumstances may mean that the benefits of treatment outweigh the risks.

Complications of chronic myeloid leukaemia

Being immunocompromised (having a weakened immune system) is a possible complication for some patients with chronic leukaemia.

There are two reasons for this:

- the lack of healthy white blood cells means your immune system is less able to fight infection
- many of the medicines used to treat chronic leukaemia can weaken the immune system

This means you are more vulnerable to developing an infection, and that any infection you have has an increased potential to cause serious complications. You may be advised to take regular doses of antibiotics to prevent infections from occurring. You should immediately report any possible symptoms of an infection to your doctor or care team because prompt treatment may be required to prevent serious complications.

Symptoms of infection include:

- high temperature (fever) of 38C (101.4F) or above
- headache
- aching muscles
- diarrhoea
- tiredness

Avoid contact with anyone who is known to have an infection, even if it is a type of infection that you were previously immune to, such as chickenpox or measles. This is because your previous immunity to these conditions will probably be suppressed (lowered).

While it is important to go outside on a regular basis, both for exercise and for your psychological wellbeing, avoid visiting crowded places and using public transport during rush hour. Also ensure that all of your vaccinations are up-to-date. Your doctor or care team will be able to advise you about this. You will be unable to have any vaccine that contains activated particles of viruses or bacteria, such as:

- the mumps, measles and rubella (MMR) vaccine
- the polio vaccine
- the oral typhoid vaccine
- the BCG vaccine (used to vaccinate against tuberculosis)
- the yellow fever vaccine
- Psychological effects of chronic leukaemia

Receiving a diagnosis of chronic leukaemia can be very distressing, particularly if it is unlikely that your condition can be cured. At first, the news may be difficult to take in. The situation can be made worse if you are confronted with the knowledge that even though your leukaemia may not currently be causing any symptoms, it could be a serious problem in later life. Having to wait many years to see how the leukaemia develops can be immensely stressful and can trigger feelings of stress, anxiety and depression. If you have been diagnosed with leukaemia, talking to a counsellor or psychiatrist (a doctor who specialises in treating mental health conditions) may help you to combat feelings of depression and anxiety. Antidepressants or medicines that help to reduce feelings of anxiety may also help you cope better with the condition.

Acute myeloid leukaemia

Leukaemia is cancer of the white blood cells. Acute leukaemia means it progresses rapidly and aggressively, and usually requires immediate treatment.

Acute leukaemia is classified according to the type of white blood cells affected. The two main types of white blood cells are:

☐ lymphocytes – mostly used to fight viral infections

☐ myeloid cells – which perform a number of different functions, such as fighting bacterial infections, defending the body against parasites and preventing the spread of tissue damage

This topic focuses on acute myeloid leukaemia (AML), which is an aggressive cancer of the myeloid cells. The following types of leukaemia are covered separately:

☐ acute lymphoblastic leukaemia

☐ chronic myeloid leukaemia

☐ chronic lymphocytic leukaemia

Signs and symptoms of AML

The symptoms of AML usually develop over a few weeks and become increasingly more severe. Symptoms can include:

- pale skin
- tiredness
- breathlessness
- frequent infections
- unusual and frequent bleeding, such as bleeding gums or nosebleeds

In more advanced cases, AML can make you extremely vulnerable to life-threatening infections or serious internal bleeding.

Seeking medical advice

You should see your doctor if you or your child have possible symptoms of AML. Although it's highly unlikely that leukaemia is the cause, these symptoms should be investigated. If your doctor thinks you may have leukaemia, they'll arrange blood tests to check your blood cell production. If the tests suggest there's a problem, you'll be urgently referred to a haematologist (a specialist in treating blood conditions) for further tests and any necessary treatment.

What causes AML?

AML occurs when specialised cells called stem cells, which are found in the bone marrow (a spongy material inside the bones), produce too many immature white blood cells. These immature cells are known as blast cells. Blast cells don't have the infection-fighting properties of healthy white blood cells, and producing too many can lead to a decrease in the number of red blood cells (which carry oxygen in the blood) and platelets (cells that help the blood to clot).

It's not clear exactly why this happens and, in most cases, there's no identifiable cause. However, a number of factors that can increase your risk of developing AML have been identified. These include:

- previous chemotherapy or radiotherapy
- exposure to very high levels of radiation (including
- previous radiotherapy treatment)
- exposure to benzene – a chemical used in manufacturing that's also found in cigarette smoke
- having an underlying blood disorder or genetic disorder, such as Down's syndrome

Who's affected

AML is a rare type of cancer, with around 2,600 people diagnosed with it each year in the UK. The risk of developing AML increases with age. It's most common in people over 65.

How AML is treated

AML is an aggressive type of cancer that can develop rapidly, so treatment usually needs to begin soon after a diagnosis is confirmed. Chemotherapy is the main treatment for AML. It's used to kill as many leukaemia cells in your body as possible and reduce the risk of the condition coming back (relapsing).In some cases, intensive chemotherapy and radiotherapy may be needed, in combination with a bone marrow or stem cell transplant, to achieve a cure. Outlook The outlook for AML largely depends on the specific type of AML you have, as well as your age and general health.

There are many subtypes of AML, which are classified according to various features – such as the specific genetic changes in the leukaemia cells. Some types of AML are more challenging to treat than others. Even if treatment is initially successful, there's still a significant risk that the condition will return at some point during the next few years. If this happens, treatment may need to be repeated. A number of medical trials have suggested that almost half of those aged under 60 diagnosed with AML will live for at least five years, and in some types of AML, such as acute promyeloid leukaemia (APML), around 85% will live for at least five years. In general, the outlook for children with AML tends to be better than that of adults diagnosed with the condition.

Symptoms of acute myeloid leukaemia

The symptoms of acute myeloid leukaemia (AML) usually

develop over a few weeks, becoming more severe as the number of immature white blood cells (blast cells) in your blood increases.

Symptoms of AML

- pale skin
- tiredness
- breathlessness
- a high temperature (fever)
- excessive sweating
- weight loss
- frequent infections
- unusual and frequent bleeding, such as bleeding gums or nosebleeds
- easily bruised skin
- flat red or purple spots on the skin (petechiae)
- bone and joint pain
- a feeling of fullness or discomfort in your tummy (abdomen), caused by swelling of the liver or spleen

In rare cases of AML, the affected cells can spread into the central nervous system. This can cause symptoms such as headaches, fits (seizures), vomiting, blurred vision and dizziness.

When to seek medical advice

See your doctor if you or your child have the symptoms listed above. Although it's highly unlikely that AML is the cause, these symptoms need to be investigated and treated promptly.

Causes of acute myeloid leukaemia

Acute myeloid leukaemia (AML) is caused by a DNA mutation in the stem cells in your bone marrow that produce red blood cells, platelets and infection-fighting white blood cells. The mutation causes the stem cells to produce many more white blood cells that are needed. The white blood cells produced are still immature, so they don't have the infection-fighting properties of fully developed white blood cells. These immature cells are known as "blast cells". As the number of immature cells increases, the amount of healthy red blood cells and platelets decrease, and it's this fall that causes many of the symptoms of leukaemia.

Increased risk

It's not known what triggers the genetic mutation in AML, although a number of different factors that can increase your risk of developing the condition have been identified.

The main risk factors for AML

Radiation exposure

Being exposed to a significant level of radiation can increase your chances of developing AML, although this usually requires exposure at very high levels. For example, rates of AML are higher in people who survived the atomic bomb explosions in Japan in 1945. In the UK, most people are unlikely to be exposed to levels of radiation high enough to cause AML. However, some people who have had radiotherapy as part of their treatment for previous cancer can be the exception.

Benzene and smoking

Exposure to the chemical benzene is a known risk factor for AML in adults. Benzene is found in petrol, and it's also used in the rubber industry, although there are strict controls to protect people from prolonged exposure. Benzene is also found in cigarette smoke, which could explain why people who smoke have an increased risk of developing AML.

Previous cancer treatment

Treatment with radiotherapy and certain chemotherapy medications for an earlier, unrelated cancer can increase your risk of developing AML many years later. Leukaemia that develops as a result of previous cancer treatment is called "secondary leukaemia" or "treatment-related leukaemia".

Blood disorders

People with certain blood disorders – such as myelodysplasia, myelofibrosis or polycythaemia vera (PCV) – have an increased risk of developing AML.

Genetic disorders

People with certain genetic disorders, including Down's syndrome and Fanconi's anaemia, have an increased risk of developing leukaemia.

Other suggested triggers

A number of other environmental factors that could trigger AML have also been suggested, including childhood vaccinations and living near a nuclear power station or a high-voltage power line. However, there's no clear evidence to suggest that these can increase your risk of developing AML.

Diagnosing acute myeloid leukaemia

In the initial stages of diagnosing acute myeloid leukaemia (AML), your doctor will check for physical signs of the condition and arrange for you to have blood tests. A high number of abnormal white blood cells, or a very low blood count in the test sample, could indicate the presence of leukaemia. If this is the case, you will be urgently referred to a haematologist (a specialist in treating blood conditions). A haematologist may carry out further blood tests, in addition to some of the tests outlined below.

Bone marrow biopsy

To confirm a diagnosis of AML, the haematologist will take a small sample of your bone marrow to examine under a microscope. This procedure is known as a bone marrow biopsy, which is usually carried out under a local anaesthetic. The haematologist will numb an area of skin at the back of your hip bone, before using a thin needle to remove a sample of liquid bone marrow. In some cases, a larger needle may also be used to remove a small amount of bone and bone marrow together. You will not feel any pain during the procedure, but you may experience some bruising and discomfort for a few days afterwards. The procedure takes around 15 minutes to complete, and you shouldn't have to stay in hospital overnight. The bone marrow sample will be checked for cancerous cells. If cancerous cells are present, the biopsy can also be used to determine the type of leukaemia you have.

Further tests

Additional tests can be used to reveal more information about the progress and extent of your AML. They can also provide insight into how the condition should be treated. These tests are described below.

Genetic testing

Genetic tests can be carried out on blood and bone marrow samples to identify the genetic makeup of the cancerous cells. There are many specific genetic variations that can occur in AML, and knowing the exact type of AML you have can help doctors make decisions about the most appropriate treatment. For example, people who have a type of AML known as acute promyelocytic leukaemia (APML) are known to respond well to a medicine called All Trans-Retinoic Acid (ATRA).

Scans

If you have AML, a computerised tomography (CT) scan, X-ray or echocardiogram (an ultrasound scan of the heart) may be used to check that your organs, such as your heart and lungs, are healthy. These tests are carried out because it's important for doctors to assess your general health before they can decide on the most appropriate treatment for you.

Lumbar puncture

In rare situations where it's thought there's a risk that AML has spread to your nervous system, a lumbar puncture may be carried out. In this procedure, a needle is used to extract a sample of cerebrospinal fluid (which surrounds and protects your spine) from your back, so it can be checked for cancerous cells. If cancerous cells are found in your nervous system, you may need to have injections of chemotherapy medication directly into your cerebrospinal fluid as part of your treatment.

Treating acute myeloid leukaemia

Acute myeloid leukaemia (AML) is an aggressive condition that develops rapidly, so treatment will usually begin a few days after a diagnosis has been confirmed. As AML is a complex condition, it's usually treated by a multidisciplinary team (MDT) – a group of different specialists working together as shown below.

Your treatment plan

Treatment for AML is often carried out in two stages:

Induction – the aim of this initial stage of treatment is to kill as many leukaemia cells in your blood and bone marrow as possible, restore your blood to proper working order and treat any symptoms you may have.

Consolidation – this stage aims to prevent the cancer returning (relapsing), by killing any remaining leukaemia cells that may be present in your body. The induction stage of treatment isn't always successful and sometimes needs to be repeated before consolidation can begin. If you have a relapse after treatment, both re-induction and consolidation may need to be carried out. This may be the same as your first treatment, although it's likely to involve different medications or a stem cell transplant.

If you are thought to have a high risk of experiencing complications of AML treatment – for example, if you are over 75 years of age or have another underlying health condition – less intensive chemotherapy treatment may be carried out. This is less likely to successfully kill all of the cancerous cells in your body, but it can help control your condition.

Induction

The initial treatment you have for AML will largely depend on whether you're fit enough to have intensive chemotherapy, or whether treatment at a lower dosage is recommended.

Intensive chemotherapy

If you can have intensive induction chemotherapy, you'll usually be given a combination of chemotherapy medication at a high dose to kill the cancerous cells in your blood and bone marrow. This stage of treatment will be carried out in hospital or in a specialist centre, as you will need very close medical and nursing supervision. You will have regular blood transfusions because your blood won't contain enough healthy blood cells. You will also be vulnerable to infection, so it's important that you're in a clean and stable environment where your health can be carefully monitored and any infection you have can be promptly treated. You may also be prescribed antibiotics to help prevent further infection. Depending on how well you respond to treatment, the induction phase can last from four weeks to a couple of months. You may be able to leave hospital and receive treatment on an outpatient basis if your symptoms improve.

For intensive treatment, the chemotherapy medications will

be injected into a thin tube that's inserted either into a blood vessel near your heart (central line) or into your arm (a peripherally inserted central catheter, or PICC). In very rare cases, chemotherapy medication may also be directly administered into your cerebrospinal fluid to kill any leukaemia cells that may have spread to your nervous system. This is done using a needle that's placed into your spine, in a similar way to a lumbar puncture.

Side effects of intensive chemotherapy for AML are common.

They can include:

- nausea
- vomiting
- diarrhoea
- loss of appetite
- sore mouth and mouth ulcers (mucositis)
- tiredness
- skin rashes
- hair loss
- infertility – which may be temporary or permanent

Most side effects should resolve once treatment has finished. Tell a member of your care team if side effects become particularly troublesome, as there are medicines that can help you cope better with certain side effects.

Non-intensive chemotherapy

If your doctors don't think you're fit enough to withstand the effects of intensive chemotherapy, they may recommend non-intensive treatment. This involves using an alternative type of chemotherapy to the standard intensive therapy, which is designed more to control leukaemia rather than cure it. The main aim of this treatment is to control the level of cancerous cells in your body and limit any symptoms you have, while reducing your risk of experiencing significant side effects of treatment. The medications used during non-intensive chemotherapy may be given through a drip into a vein, by mouth or by injection under the skin, and can often be given on an outpatient basis.

All Trans-Retinoic Acid (ATRA)

If you have the sub-type of AML known as acute promyelocytic leukaemia, you will usually be given capsules of a medicine called ATRA, in addition to chemotherapy. ATRA works by changing the immature white blood cells (blast cells) into mature healthy cells, and can reduce symptoms very quickly. Side effects of ATRA can include headaches, nausea, bone pain, and dry mouth, skin and eyes.

Consolidation

If induction is successful, the next stage of treatment will be consolidation. This often involves receiving regular injections of chemotherapy medication that are usually given on an outpatient basis, which means that you won't have to stay in hospital overnight. However, you may need some short stays in hospital if your symptoms suddenly get worse or if you develop an infection.

The consolidation phase of treatment lasts several months.

Other treatments

Many other treatments are used for AML, as described below.

Radiotherapy

Radiotherapy involves using high doses of controlled radiation to kill cancerous cells. There are two main reasons why radiotherapy is usually used to treat AML:

- to prepare the body for a bone marrow or stem cell transplant
- to treat advanced cases that have spread to the nervous system or brain, although this is uncommon

Side effects of radiotherapy can include hair loss, nausea and fatigue. The side effects should pass once your course of radiotherapy has been completed.

Bone marrow and stem cell transplants

If chemotherapy doesn't work, a possible alternative treatment option is a bone marrow or stem cell transplant. Before transplantation can take place, the person receiving the transplant will need to have intensive high-dose chemotherapy and possibly radiotherapy to destroy the cells in their bone marrow. The donated stem cells are given through a tube into a blood vessel, in a similar way to chemotherapy medication. This process can put an enormous amount of strain on the body and cause significant side effects and potential complications, so you'll usually need to stay in hospital for a few weeks. Transplantations have better outcomes if the donor has the same tissue type as the person receiving the donation. The best candidate to provide a donation is usually a brother or sister with the same tissue type. Transplantations are most successful when they're carried out on children and young people, or older people who are otherwise in good health, and when there's a suitable donor, such as a brother or sister.

Azacitidine

Azacitidine is a possible alternative treatment for adults with AML who cannot have a stem cell transplant. It's recommended by the National Institute for Health and Care Excellence (NICE) for use in certain circumstances – for example, depending on the characteristics of the person's blood and bone marrow. Azacitidine is a chemotherapy medication that's given by injection under the skin. It interferes with the growth of cancer cells and destroys them, and also helps bone marrow to produce normal blood cells.

Clinical trials and newer unlicensed treatments

In the UK, a number of clinical trials are currently underway that aim to find the best way of treating AML. Clinical trials are studies that use new and experimental techniques to see how well they work in treating, and possibly curing, AML. As part of your treatment, your care team may suggest taking part in a clinical trial to help researchers learn more about the best way to treat your AML, and AML in general. Search for clinical trials for AML. If you take part in a clinical trial, you may be offered medication that isn't licensed for use in the UK and isn't normally available. However, there's no guarantee that the techniques being studied in the clinical trial will work better than current treatments.

Complications of acute myeloid leukaemia

If you have acute myeloid leukaemia (AML), you may experience a number of complications. These can be caused by the condition itself, although they can also occur as a side effect of treatment. Some of the main complications associated with AML are outlined below.

Weakened immune system

Having a weakened immune system – being

immunocompromised – is a common complication of AML.Even if your blood is restored to normal working order with treatment, many of the medications that are used to treat AML can temporarily weaken your immune system. This means you're more vulnerable to developing an infection, and any infection you develop could be more serious than usual. Complications arising from infection are the leading cause of death in people with AML. However, if treated early, nearly all infections respond to appropriate treatment.

Therefore, you may be advised to:

- take regular doses of antibiotics to prevent bacterial infections
- maintain good personal and dental hygiene
- avoid contact with anyone who's known to have an infection – even if it's a type of infection that you were previously immune to, such as chickenpox or measles

check with your doctor to ensure that all of your vaccinations are up to date, although you won't be able to have any vaccine that contains "live" viruses or bacteria, such as the shingles vaccine and MMR vaccine (against measles, mumps and rubella) Report any possible symptoms of an infection to your treatment unit immediately because prompt treatment may be needed to prevent complications.

Symptoms of an infection can include:

- a high temperature (fever)
- a headache
- aching muscles
- diarrhoea
- tiredness
- Bleeding

If you have AML, you'll bleed and bruise more easily due to the low levels of platelets (clot-forming cells) in your blood. Bleeding may also be excessive. People with advanced AML are more vulnerable to excessive bleeding inside their body, which is the second most common cause of death in people with the condition.

Serious bleeding can occur:

- inside the skull (intracranial haemorrhage) – causing symptoms such as a severe headache, stiff neck, vomiting and confusion
- inside the lungs (pulmonary haemorrhage) – causing symptoms such as coughing up blood, breathing difficulties and a bluish skin tone (cyanosis)
- inside the stomach (gastrointestinal haemorrhage) – causing symptoms such as vomiting blood and passing stools (faeces) that are very dark or tar-like in colour

Infertility

Many of the treatments that are used to treat AML can cause infertility. This is often temporary, but in some cases can be permanent. People who are particularly at risk of permanent infertility, are those who have received high doses of chemotherapy and radiotherapy in preparation for a bone marrow or stem cell transplant. Your treatment team can give a good estimation of the risk of infertility in your specific circumstances. It may be possible to guard against any risk of infertility before you begin your treatment. For example, men can have their sperm samples stored. Similarly, women can have eggs or fertilised embryos stored, which can then be placed back into their womb, following treatment. However, as AML is an aggressive condition that develops rapidly, there may not always be time to do this before treatment needs to start.

Acute lymphoblastic leukaemia (ALL)

Acute lymphoblastic leukaemia (ALL) is a type of blood cancer that starts from young white blood cells called lymphocytes in the bone marrow. Adults and children can get it but it is most often diagnosed in younger people. Chemotherapy is the main treatment. Some people need to have a stem cell transplant.

What is acute lymphoblastic leukaemia (ALL)

Acute lymphoblastic leukaemia (ALL) is a type of blood cancer. It starts from young white blood cells called lymphocytes in the bone marrow. The bone marrow is the soft inner part of the bones, where new blood cells are made. ALL usually develops quickly over days or weeks. It is the most common type of leukaemia to affect children but can also affect adults.

How common is ALL?

Acute lymphoblastic leukaemia is rare. Around 790 people are diagnosed with ALL in the UK each year. ALL is most often diagnosed in children, teenagers and young adults. The age group with the highest incidence is young children aged 0 - 4 years.

What happens in ALL

The word acute means that the leukaemia can develop quickly. This is because the lymphocytes are growing and dividing much quicker than usual. These abnormal cells build up in the blood.

The leukaemia cells can spread into other parts of the body, including the:

☐ lymph nodes

☐ liver

- spleen
- central nervous system (brain and spinal cord)
- testicles

The leukaemia cells can build up in the lymph nodes, bone marrow and spleen and make them bigger. If it wasn't treated acute leukaemia would cause death within a few weeks or months. But treatments work well for most people with ALL.

Blood cells and ALL

To understand how and why leukaemia affects you as it does, it helps to know how you make blood cells. Your body makes blood cells in the bone marrow. The bone marrow is the soft inner part of your bones. You make blood cells in a controlled way, as your body needs them.

All blood cells start as the same type of cell, called a stem cell. This stem cell then develops into:

- lymphoid stem cells, which become white blood cells called lymphocytes
- myeloid stem cells, which become white blood cells called monocytes and neutrophils (granulocytes), red blood cells and platelets

The diagram helps explain this:

C:\Users\CC LEEDS\Downloads\fffffff.png

In acute lymphoblastic leukaemia, the bone marrow makes

too many lymphocytes. These lymphocytes are not fully developed and are not able to work normally.

C:\Users\CC LEEDS\Downloads\cccccccc.png

Diagram showing which cell ALL starts in

Types of leukaemia

There are several types and subtypes of leukaemia. The name of the leukaemia you have depends on:

- how quickly it develops
- the type of white blood cells it affects

Doctors divide leukaemia into two main groups, acute and chronic. Acute leukaemia develops very quickly. Chronic leukaemia tends to develop slowly, usually over months or years without causing many symptoms.

Doctors divide these groups further, depending on the type of white blood cell they affect.

In acute leukaemia:

- acute myeloid leukaemia (AML) affects myeloid cells
- acute lymphoblastic leukaemia (ALL) affects lymphoid cells

In chronic leukaemia:

- chronic myeloid leukaemia (CML) affects myeloid cells
- chronic lymphocytic leukaemia (CLL) affects lymphoid cells

How leukaemia can affect you

White blood cells help fight infection. But if your body makes abnormal white blood cells, they don't work properly. So you are more likely to get infections and find it difficult to get rid of them. Too many white blood cells can overcrowd the bone marrow. So there isn't enough space for other types of blood cells. This can cause a lower than normal number of red blood cells and platelets. Having too few red blood cells makes you tired and breathless (anaemic). You can have bleeding problems such as nosebleeds, if you don't have enough platelets. Abnormal white blood cells can build up in parts of the lymphatic system, such as the spleen and lymph nodes, making them bigger. They might build up in the liver. This can make your tummy (abdomen) swell and feel uncomfortable.

Symptoms

Many symptoms of ALL are vague and non-specific. You may feel as if you have flu. These symptoms are caused by too many abnormal white blood cells and not enough normal white cells, red cells and platelets. Most people with one or more of these symptoms don't have leukaemia. But it's important to get any symptoms checked out by your doctor.

General weakness

☐ You might feel weaker than normal.

- Feeling tired (fatigue)
- You might feel more tired than normal, even if you're getting a good night's sleep.
- High temperature (fever)
- You might have a high temperature or feel feverish.

Frequent infections

You might pick up infections such as coughs and colds easily. Or you might find that the infections last a long time and are difficult to shake off. This is because you don't have enough healthy white blood cells to fight bacteria or viruses.

You might have:

- nosebleeds
- bleeding gums when you clean your teeth
- very heavy periods
- small dark red spots on your skin
- blood in your wee (urine) or poo (stool)
- You might find you are bruising more easily than normal.
- Weight loss
- You might lose weight even if you haven't changed your diet.

Swollen lymph nodes

Your lymph nodes (glands) might feel swollen when you

touch them. You have lymph nodes in lots of places in your body. They might feel swollen in:

- ☐ your neck
- ☐ under your armpit
- ☐ in your groin

Pain in your bones or joints

You might feel pain in your bones or joints. This might be a dull ache or more of a stabbing pain. It might be worse at different times of the day. Too many abnormal white blood cells collecting in the bones, joints or lymph nodes may cause pain and swelling.

Feeling short of breath (breathlessness)

You might feel breathless when doing your normal day to day activities or from climbing a short flight of stairs. This could be because you do not have enough red blood cells.

Feeling full in your tummy (abdomen)

You might have a feeling of fullness or discomfort in your tummy (abdomen). This can happen if your liver or spleen are swollen.

Pale skin

You might look paler or more 'washed out' than normal.

When to see your doctor

You should get any of these symptoms checked by your doctor. But remember, they can all be caused by other medical conditions. Most people with these symptoms don't have leukaemia.

Symptoms of T cell ALL

A type of leukaemia called T cell ALL can cause swollen lymph nodes in the centre of your chest. It might make the thymus gland in your upper chest bigger. The swollen nodes or thymus gland may press on the windpipe, causing breathlessness and coughing. They can also press on the veins carrying blood from the head. This causes pressure in the blood vessels and makes the face, neck and arms swell and go red. This is called superior vena cava obstruction (SVCO).

Getting diagnosed

You usually start by seeing your doctor if you have symptoms. Your doctor will examine you and might arrange blood tests. If the results show signs of acute lymphoblastic leukaemia (ALL) they will refer you straight away to see a specialist.

Risks and causes

Your risk of developing cancer depends on many things including environmental, lifestyle and genetic factors. Anything that can increase or decrease your risk of cancer is called a risk factor. We don't know what causes most cases of acute lymphoblastic leukaemia (ALL). But there are some factors that may increase your risk of developing it. Having one or more risk factors doesn't mean that you will definitely get leukaemia.

Risk factors for ALL include:

- Ionising radiation exposure
- Exposure to benzene
- Smoking
- Genetic conditions
- Past chemotherapy
- Viruses
- Electromagnetic fields
- House painting exposure
- Weakened immunity

Other possible causes

Stories about potential causes are often in the media and it isn't always clear which ideas are supported by evidence.

There might be things you have heard of that we haven't included here. This is because either there is no evidence about them or it is less clear.

Risk factors for ALL and explanation

Ionising radiation exposure

We have known for a long time that exposure to very high levels of ionising radiation increases acute leukaemia risk. For example, people exposed to the atomic bomb explosions in Japan at the end of World War 2 had higher rates of leukaemia. A 20 year study has followed up workers who helped clean up after the Chernobyl nuclear power plant accident in 1986. It shows that even at low doses of ionising radiation there is an increased risk of all types of leukaemia. Some people worry that childhood x-rays cause leukaemia in children. A large study found there is very little evidence of any increase in risk, except in a type of leukaemia that is rare in children, called pre B cell ALL (or pre B ALL). But the researchers say that even this could be a chance finding and not a real risk increase. There is some evidence that x-rays during pregnancy could increase the risk of childhood leukaemia. So doctors avoid x-rays for pregnant women whenever possible. CT scans and radiotherapy treatment also use ionising radiation. Research has also suggested that in children this could increase the risk of developing leukaemia in the future. However, it's important to note that doctors make sure the benefits of having the test or treatment outweighs the risks.

Exposure to benzene

Exposure to a chemical called benzene at work can increase the risk of developing ALL. Exposure to benzene may occur in petrol, chemical, pharmaceutical and rubber industries. Benzene is also used in shoe production and the printing industry. The higher the level of exposure over many years, the greater the risk. There is benzene in traffic pollution but the levels are likely to be too low to increase leukaemia risk.

Smoking

Cigarette smoke contains lots of harmful chemicals (including benzene) that can cause at least 15 types of cancer in adults, including leukaemia. Studies have also shown that parents who smoke may increase the risk of leukaemia in their children. This could include smoking by the father in the time before conception.

Genetic conditions

Certain rare, inherited conditions can increase the risk of acute leukaemia, including:

- Down's syndrome
- Fanconi anaemia
- ataxia telangiectasia
- Bloom syndrome

Past chemotherapy

People who have had certain chemotherapy drugs in the past have a slightly increased risk of developing leukaemia some years later. The risk depends on how much treatment you had. Some of the drugs include:

- etoposide with cisplatin and bleomycin
- thiotepa
- busulfan
- chlorambucil
- melphalan

It's important to remember that this risk is still very small compared to the risk to your health if the cancer had not been treated.

Viruses

We know that a virus called HTLV-1 (human T cell leukaemia virus) increases the risk of developing a rare type of adult T cell leukaemia. HTLV-1 is a very rare virus in the UK, and most people who carry the virus do not develop cancer because of it. The virus can spread through blood (sharing needles), bodily fluids (unprotected sex) and from mother to baby (mainly through breastfeeding).

Exposure to infection in childhood

Children may have a slightly increased risk of ALL if they

do not come across common infections from birth, but are exposed to them later in life. Researchers continue to look into this along with other factors like genetics.

Electromagnetic fields

You may read in the press from time to time that some people are concerned about power lines and risk of cancer. Power lines produce high levels of 'low frequency electromagnetic radiation' (EMR). Although some studies seem to suggest that exposure to very high levels of EMR could increase childhood leukaemia risk, the findings are not very clear. We don't really know if the childhood leukaemia in these studies was actually caused by low frequency EMR. It could be due to some other common factors, or even chance. In 2018, a large international study of overhead power lines and child leukaemia found no association. This was true even for children living within 50 metres of a power line.

House painting exposure

Studies have suggested a slightly higher risk of childhood ALL after high exposure to house painting. But the findings are not conclusive and we need more studies to back up this finding.

Weakened immunity

An overview study (combined analysis) looked at published

research into people with HIV or AIDS, or people treated with medicines that lower immunity after an organ transplant. The researchers found that these people have a risk of leukaemia that is double or triple that of people without these factors.

Treatment

The main treatment for acute lymphoblastic leukaemia (ALL) is chemotherapy. You usually have steroids as well. You might also have treatment with a targeted cancer drug. Some people will need a stem cell transplant.

Treatment options

A team of doctors and other professionals discuss the best treatment and care for you. They are called a multi-disciplinary team (MDT).

Your MDT might include:

- blood cancer specialists called consultant haematologists
- haematology nurse specialists, also called clinical nurse specialists (CNS)
- dietitians
- doctors specialising in reporting bone marrow or lymph node biopsies (haemopathologists)
- doctors specialising in reporting x-rays and scans (radiologists)

- doctors specialising in diagnosing and controlling infection (microbiologists)
- social workers
- symptom control specialists called palliative care doctors and nurses
- pharmacists

Your MDT will discuss your treatment, its benefits and the possible side effects with you. Your treatment will depend on:

- the type of leukaemia you have
- your age, general health and level of fitness
- if you have gene changes (mutations) in the leukaemia cells

The main treatments for ALL

Most people with ALL start treatment quickly after diagnosis. The main treatment is chemotherapy.

Apart from chemotherapy other treatments for ALL include:

- steroids
- targeted cancer drugs
- radiotherapy
- growth factors
- stem cell or bone marrow transplants

Other treatment

You might need other treatments to support you while you have your main leukaemia treatment. This might be because you have an infection or to help with the side effects of treatment. These include:

- anti-sickness medicines
- painkillers
- blood or platelet transfusions
- medicines to protect your kidneys
- antibiotics
- fluid through a drip to keep you hydrated

Phases of treatment

Doctors divide treatment for ALL into 3 different phases. The treatment usually takes 2 to 3 year's altogether. The maintenance therapy phase takes up most of this time.

Getting rid of ALL (remission induction)

The aim of the induction phase is to destroy the leukaemia cells. This is called complete remission (CR). It means there is no sign of the leukaemia in your blood or bone marrow. The main treatment is chemotherapy. If you have Philadelphia positive ALL you also have a targeted cancer drug called imatinib.

Treatment to stop ALL coming back (consolidation or intensification therapy)

Consolidation therapy is when the treatment is made stronger. The aim is to get rid of any leukaemia cells that might still be there and to stop it from coming back. You might have:

- more chemotherapy
- a transplant using stem cells from someone else (donor)
- a transplant with your own blood stem cells, but this is rare
- Read about having a stem cell transplant
- Keeping ALL away long term (maintenance therapy)

The last phase of ALL treatment is maintenance therapy. It helps to keep the leukaemia in remission. This is usually chemotherapy and short courses of steroids.

Treating ALL that comes back or resists treatment

Sometimes tests still find leukaemia cells in the bone marrow while you're having treatment. This means the leukaemia isn't responding to the drugs you're having. It's called resistant or refractory leukaemia.

Your doctor may recommend you have:

- more chemotherapy using different drugs
- a targeted cancer drug

- treatment as part of a clinical trial

Leukaemia that comes back after treatment is called relapsed leukaemia. Treatment depends on:

- certain features of the leukaemia cells
- how long you were in remission
- your age, general health and level of fitness
- what treatment you had before

Your doctor may recommend you have:

- chemotherapy
- a targeted cancer drug
- taking part in a clinical trial
- a stem cell transplant

Clinical trials

You often have treatment for ALL as part of a clinical trial. Doctors and researchers do trials to make existing treatments better and develop new treatments.

Phases of treatment

Treatment for acute lymphoblastic leukaemia (ALL) is divided into 3 phases. These are:

- remission induction
- consolidation therapy
- maintenance therapy

Treatment for ALL usually takes between 2 and 3 years. The maintenance phase of treatment takes up most of this time.

Getting rid of ALL (remission induction)

Aim of the induction phase

The aim of the induction phase is to destroy the leukaemia cells. If there is no sign of leukaemia in your blood and bone marrow after treatment it is called a complete remission (CR).

What treatment to expect

You start treatment quite quickly after being diagnosed. The main treatment is chemotherapy. You have several chemotherapy drugs over a few days. Chemotherapy kills off many of your healthy bone marrow cells as well as the leukaemia cells. So you need to stay in hospital for about a month until you have recovered. There are different combinations of drugs your doctors might use. You usually start taking steroids for up to a week before you start chemotherapy. This starts to get rid of some of the leukaemia cells while your doctor gets all your test results and plans your treatment.

Steroids

You also take medicine and have fluid through a drip to help protect your kidneys. You take antibiotics if you have an infection. You might also need blood or platelet transfusions depending on your blood test results. If you have Philadelphia positive ALL you have a targeted cancer drug called imatinib (Glivec) as well as chemotherapy. You take this as a tablet every day.

Chemotherapy into the spine

Leukaemia cells can sometimes travel to the brain and spinal cord (the central nervous system, CNS). So as part of your induction treatment you have chemotherapy and possibly a steroid into the fluid that circulates around the spinal cord and brain. This is called intrathecal chemotherapy. It treats leukaemia cells that are in the CNS. Or you have it to prevent leukaemia cells spreading to the CNS (CNS prophylaxis). Having this treatment is like having a lumbar puncture.

What happens next

A specialist doctor checks a sample of your bone marrow under a microscope after you have finished the induction phase. This is to check how well the treatment has worked. You move on to the next phase of treatment if you are in remission (consolidation). If you're not in remission you usually have more chemotherapy.

Treatment to stop ALL coming back (consolidation therapy)

Aim of consolidation therapy

Consolidation therapy is when the treatment is made stronger. Your doctor might also call it the intensification phase. The aim is to get rid of any leukaemia cells that might still be there and to stop it from coming back.

This phase of treatment might take a few months.

What treatment to expect

You have one of the following:

- ☐ more chemotherapy
- ☐ a donor transplant
- ☐ a transplant with your own blood stem cells, but this is rare

A donor transplant means having bone marrow or stem cells from someone else. This is called an allogeneic transplant or allograft. Before the transplant you have either high dose chemotherapy or radiotherapy to the whole body (total body irradiation, TBI) and high dose chemotherapy. The consolidation treatment you have depends on many factors. These include:

- whether your lumbar puncture tests show leukaemia cells in the fluid around your brain and spinal cord
- whether your leukaemia is completely in remission
- how many times you had chemotherapy before your leukaemia went into remission
- whether you developed leukaemia after treatment for another cancer
- your general health and level of fitness

What happens next

You usually start maintenance therapy after finishing your consolidation therapy. If you have a transplant you won't need maintenance therapy. Your transplant team follows you up very closely once you are well enough to go home.

Keeping ALL away long term (maintenance therapy)

The last phase of ALL treatment is maintenance therapy. It helps to keep the leukaemia in remission.

What to expect

You usually have low dose chemotherapy and short courses of steroids for around 2 years. You also have intrathecal chemotherapy. You have your treatment in cycles, also known as blocks. You see your doctor every few months to check how you are getting on and to keep an eye on your blood counts. Sometimes you may need blood transfusions or antibiotics if you have an infection.

What happens next

Your doctor follows you up closely after you finish maintenance therapy. You have regular blood tests and meet with your doctor to see how you are. You can still contact your specialist nurse between appointments if you have any problems.

Clinical trials

Your doctor may ask you to take part in a clinical trial as part of your treatment. Doctors and researchers do trials to:

- improve treatment
- make existing treatments better
- develop new treatments

Talk to your doctor or clinical nurse specialist if you are interested in joining a clinical trial.

Chemotherapy for ALL

Chemotherapy uses anti-cancer (cytotoxic) drugs to destroy cancer cells. The drugs circulate throughout the body in the bloodstream. Chemotherapy is the main treatment for acute lymphoblastic leukaemia (ALL). You have several different chemotherapy drugs, usually with a steroid. You may have treatment as part of a clinical trial. Your exact treatment depends on a number of factors but you can usually divide it into phases.

Phases of treatment for ALL

Your treatment is in 3 phases:
- getting rid of ALL (remission induction)
- treatment to stop ALL coming back (consolidation)
- keeping ALL away long term (maintenance)
- Getting rid of ALL (remission induction)

Aim of the induction phase

The aim of the induction phase is to destroy the leukaemia cells. If there is no sign of leukaemia in your blood and bone marrow after treatment it is called a complete remission (CR).

What treatment to expect

You start treatment quite quickly after being diagnosed. The main treatment is chemotherapy. You have several chemotherapy drugs over a few days. Chemotherapy kills off many of your healthy bone marrow cells as well as the leukaemia cells. So you need to stay in hospital for about a month until you have recovered. There are different combinations of drugs your doctors might use. You usually start taking steroids for up to a week before you start chemotherapy. This starts to get rid of some of the leukaemia cells while your doctor gets all your test results and plans your treatment.

Steroids

You also take medicine and have fluid through a drip to help protect your kidneys. You take antibiotics if you have an infection. You might also need blood or platelet transfusions depending on your blood test results. If you have Philadelphia positive ALL you have a targeted cancer drug called imatinib (Glivec) as well as chemotherapy. You take this as a tablet every day.

Chemotherapy into the spine

Leukaemia cells can sometimes travel to the brain and spinal cord (the central nervous system, CNS). So as part of your induction treatment you have chemotherapy and possibly a steroid into the fluid that circulates around the spinal cord and brain. This is called intrathecal chemotherapy. It treats leukaemia cells that are in the CNS. Or you have it to prevent leukaemia cells spreading to the CNS (CNS prophylaxis).Having this treatment is like having a lumbar puncture.

What happens next

A specialist doctor checks a sample of your bone marrow under a microscope after you have finished the induction phase. This is to check how well the treatment has worked. You move on to the next phase of treatment if you are in remission (consolidation). If you're not in remission you usually have more chemotherapy.

Treatment to stop ALL coming back (consolidation)

The second phase of treatment is called the consolidation or intensification phase. The aim is to destroy any leukaemia cells that may still be in your blood or bone marrow but can't be picked up on tests. It reduces the risk of the leukaemia coming back. This phase of treatment usually lasts several months. There are different types of consolidation treatment. You might have high doses of one of the chemotherapy drugs that you had as part of your induction treatment. You might be able to have some of this treatment as an outpatient.

A common chemotherapy combination includes:

- doxorubicin
- asparaginase
- methotrexate
- cytarabine

Some people have high dose chemotherapy and radiotherapy followed by a stem cell or bone marrow transplant.

Keeping ALL away, long term (maintenance)

The aim of maintenance treatment is to help keep the leukaemia in remission. You have more chemotherapy, but in lower doses than in the other phases of treatment. You also have steroids. The drugs that you are likely to have during maintenance include:

- methotrexate
- vincristine
- mercaptopurine
- prednisolone (a steroid)
- intrathecal chemotherapy

The maintenance phase lasts for about 2 years. You usually have this as an outpatient, and most people can go back to work, school or college during this phase.

How you have chemotherapy

You can have treatment through a thin short tube (a cannula) that goes into a vein in your arm each time you have treatment. Or you might have it through a long line: a central line, a PICC line or a Portacath. These are long plastic tubes that give the drug into a large vein in your chest. The tube stays in place throughout the course of treatment.

Side effects

Treatment for ALL can cause side effects. These include:
- a drop in your blood cell counts
- feeling and being sick
- a sore mouth and mouth ulcers
- diarrhoea
- tiredness
- loss of fertility
- hair loss

Contact your doctor or nurse immediately if you have signs of infection, including a temperature above 37.5C or below 36C, or generally feel unwell. Infections can make you very unwell very quickly.

Clinical trials

Your doctor may offer you treatment as part of a clinical trial.

When at home

Chemotherapy for ALL can be difficult to cope with. Tell your doctor or nurse about any problems or side effects that you have. Your nurse will give you telephone numbers to call if you have any problems at home.

Chemotherapy drugs

Chemotherapy is the main treatment for acute lymphoblastic leukaemia. You usually have several chemotherapy drugs, often with steroids. Find out about the different types of chemotherapy drugs doctors may use for the treatment of ALL, and the possible side effects.

Amsacrine (Amsidine, m-AMSA)

Find out what amsacrine is, how you have it and other important information about having amsacrine. Amsacrine is a chemotherapy drug and is also called amsidine or m-AMSA.

It is used to treat some types of:

☐ lymphoma

☐ acute adult leukaemia

How it works

One of the ways amsacrine works is by blocking an enzyme called topoisomerase 2. If this enzyme is blocked the cell's DNA gets tangled up and the cell can't split into 2 new cancer cells. Amsacrine also works as an alkylating agent. This is a type of chemotherapy drug that works by sticking to one of the cancer cell's DNA strands.

How you have it

You have amsacrine into your bloodstream (intravenously).

It is a red liquid.

Drugs into your bloodstream

You have the treatment through a drip into your arm or hand. A nurse puts a small tube (a cannula) into one of your veins and connects the drip to it. You might need a central line. This is a long plastic tube that gives the drugs into a large vein, either in your chest or through a vein in your arm. It stays in while you're having treatment, which may be for a few months.

When you have it

You usually have chemotherapy as a course of several cycles of treatment. You may have amsacrine daily for between 3 and 5 days, every 3 to 4 weeks. The chemotherapy drip usually takes an hour.

Tests

You have blood tests before and during your treatment. They check your levels of blood cells and other substances in the blood. They also check how well your liver and kidneys are working.

Other medicines, food and drink

Cancer drugs can interact with some other medicines and herbal products. Tell your doctor or pharmacist about any medicines you are taking. This includes vitamins, herbal supplements and over the counter remedies.

Pregnancy and contraception

This treatment might harm a baby developing in the womb. It is important not to become pregnant or father a child while you're having treatment and for a few months afterwards. Talk to your doctor or nurse about effective contraception before starting treatment.

Fertility

You may not be able to become pregnant or father a child after treatment with this drug. Talk to your doctor before starting treatment if you think you may want to have a baby in the future. Men may be able to store sperm before starting treatment. Women may be able to store eggs or ovarian tissue but this is rare.

Breastfeeding

Don't breastfeed during this treatment because the drug may come through into your breast milk.

Treatment for other conditions

Always tell other doctors, nurses, pharmacists or dentists that you are having this treatment if you need treatment for anything else, including teeth problems.

Immunisations

Don't have immunisations with live vaccines while you're having treatment and for up to 12 months afterwards. The length of time depends on the treatment you are having. Ask your doctor or pharmacist how long you should avoid live vaccinations. In the UK, live vaccines include rubella, mumps, measles, BCG, yellow fever and the shingles vaccine (Zostavax).

You can:

- have other vaccines, but they might not give you as much protection as usual
- have the flu vaccine (as an injection)
- be in contact with other people who have had live vaccines as injections
- Avoid close contact with people who have recently had live vaccines taken by mouth (oral vaccines) such as oral polio or the typhoid vaccine.

This also includes the rotavirus vaccine given to babies. The virus is in the baby's poo for up to 2 weeks and could make you ill. So avoid changing their nappies for 2 weeks after their vaccination if possible. Or wear disposable gloves and wash your hands well afterwards. You should also avoid close contact with children who have had the flu vaccine nasal spray if your immune system is severely weakened.

Asparaginase (Crisantaspase, Erwinase)

What is Asparaginase?

Asparaginase is a chemotherapy drug used to treat acute lymphoblastic leukaemia (ALL). It can also be used to treat some other blood disorders. It also has the names Erwinase, Crisantaspase or L-asparaginase. One form of asparaginase is made from a type of bacteria called escherichia coli.

Another form of asparaginase is made from Erwinia chrysanthemi bacteria.

How it works

Asparaginase is an enzyme that breaks down a chemical in cancer cells. The cells need this chemical to make protein to create new cells. So asparaginase stops the cancer cells from dividing and growing.

How you have it

You may have asparaginase as an injection into a vein (IV) or as an injection just under the skin. But you are more likely to have it as a series of injections into a muscle in your arm or leg (IM). Your doctor will decide what dose you need, how often you will have it, and how long you need it for. It varies according to your body weight, your specific type of leukaemia and how quickly it works.

Into your bloodstream

You have the treatment through a drip into your arm or hand. A nurse puts a small tube (a cannula) into one of your veins and connects the drip to it. You might need a central line. This is a long plastic tube that gives the drugs into a large vein, either in your chest or through a vein in your arm. It stays in while you're having treatment, which may be for a few months.

Injection into a muscle

This is called an intramuscular injection. You might have stinging or a dull ache for a short time after this type of injection, but they are not usually very painful.

Tests

You have blood tests before and during your treatment. They check your levels of blood cells and other substances in the blood. They also check how well your liver and kidneys are working.

Side effects

Other medicines, foods and drink

Cancer drugs can interact with some other medicines and herbal products. Tell your doctor or pharmacist about any medicines you are taking. This includes vitamins, herbal supplements and over the counter remedies.

Pregnancy and contraception

This treatment might harm a baby developing in the womb. It is important not to become pregnant or father a child while you're having treatment and for a few months afterwards. Talk to your doctor or nurse about effective contraception before starting treatment.

Fertility

You may not be able to become pregnant or father a child after treatment with this drug. Talk to your doctor before starting treatment if you think you may want to have a baby in the future. Men may be able to store sperm before starting treatment. Women may be able to store eggs or ovarian tissue but this is rare.

Breastfeeding

Don't breastfeed during this treatment because the drug may come through into your breast milk.

Immunisations

Don't have immunisations with live vaccines while you're having treatment and for up to 12 months afterwards. The length of time depends on the treatment you are having. Ask your doctor or pharmacist how long you should avoid live vaccinations. In the UK, live vaccines include rubella, mumps, measles, BCG, yellow fever and the shingles vaccine (Zostavax).

You can:

- have other vaccines, but they might not give you as much protection as usual
- have the flu vaccine (as an injection)
- be in contact with other people who have had live vaccines as injections
- Avoid close contact with people who have recently had live vaccines taken by mouth (oral vaccines) such as oral polio or the typhoid vaccine.

This also includes the rotavirus vaccine given to babies. The virus is in the baby's poo for up to 2 weeks and could make you ill. So avoid changing their nappies for 2 weeks after their vaccination if possible. Or wear disposable gloves and wash your hands well afterwards. You should also avoid close contact with children who have had the flu vaccine nasal spray if your immune system is severely weakened.

Glucose and asparaginase

Asparaginase contains some glucose. Let your doctor know if you are diabetic. You may need to monitor your glucose levels more often.

Cyclophosphamide

Cyclophosphamide (pronounced sigh-clo-fos-fah-mide) is a chemotherapy drug. It is a treatment for several different types of cancer. You can have cyclophosphamide on its own, or in combination with other chemotherapy drugs.

How it works

Cyclophosphamide belongs to a group of drugs called alkylating agents. It works by sticking to one of the cancer cell's DNA strands. DNA is the genetic code that is in the heart of all animal and plant cells. It controls everything the cell does. The cell cannot then divide into 2 new cells.

How you have it

You have cyclophosphamide into your bloodstream (intravenously) or as tablets that you swallow whole, with a glass of water. Don't chew or break the tablets and, if possible, take the tablets in the morning.

Drugs into your bloodstream

You have the treatment through a drip into your arm or hand. A nurse puts a small tube (a cannula) into one of your veins and connects the drip to it. You might need a central line. This is a long plastic tube that gives the drugs into a large vein, either in your chest or through a vein in your arm. It stays in while you're having treatment, which may be for a few months.

Taking your tablets

- You must take tablets according to the instructions your doctor or pharmacist gives you.
- You should take the right dose, not more or less.
- Talk to your specialist or advice line before you stop taking a cancer drug.

When you have it

You have cyclophosphamide as cycles of treatment. Your plan depends on the type of cancer you have. And whether you're having cyclophosphamide on its own or with other chemotherapy drugs. Your doctor or nurse will tell you how often and when you will have it.

Tests

You have blood tests before and during your treatment. They check your levels of blood cells and other substances in the blood. They also check how well your liver and kidneys are working.

Other medicines, foods and drink

Cancer drugs can interact with some other medicines and herbal products. Tell your doctor or pharmacist about any medicines you are taking. This includes vitamins, herbal supplements and over the counter remedies. You should not eat grapefruit or drink grapefruit juice when you are taking this drug because it can react with the drug.

Alcohol

Check with your doctor to see if drinking alcohol may harm you while having this treatment.

Pregnancy and contraception

This treatment may harm a baby developing in the womb. It is important not to become pregnant or father a child while you are having treatment. Talk to your doctor or nurse about effective contraception before starting treatment. Women must not become pregnant for at least a year after the end of treatment. Men should not father a child for at least 6 months after treatment.

Loss of fertility

You may not be able to become pregnant or father a child after treatment with this drug. Talk to your doctor before starting treatment if you think you may want to have a baby in the future. Men may be able to store sperm before starting treatment. Women may be able to store eggs or ovarian tissue but this is rare.

Breastfeeding

Don't breastfeed during this treatment because the drug may come through into your breast milk.

Treatment for other conditions

Always tell other doctors, nurses, pharmacists or dentists that you're having this treatment if you need treatment for anything else, including teeth problems.

Immunisations

Don't have immunisations with live vaccines while you're having treatment and for up to 12 months afterwards. The length of time depends on the treatment you are having. Ask your doctor or pharmacist how long you should avoid live vaccinations. In the UK, live vaccines include rubella, mumps, measles, BCG, yellow fever and the shingles vaccine (Zostavax).

You can:

- have other vaccines, but they might not give you as much protection as usual
- have the flu vaccine (as an injection)
- be in contact with other people who have had live vaccines as injections
- Avoid close contact with people who have recently had live vaccines taken by mouth (oral vaccines) such as oral polio or the typhoid vaccine.

This also includes the rotavirus vaccine given to babies. The virus is in the baby's poo for up to 2 weeks and could make you ill. So avoid changing their nappies for 2 weeks after their vaccination if possible. Or wear disposable gloves and wash your hands well afterwards. You should also avoid close contact with children who have had the flu vaccine nasal spray if your immune system is severely weakened.

Cytarabine (Ara C, cytosine arabinoside)

Cytarabine is, how you have it and other important information about having cytarabine. Cytarabine, sometimes called cytosine arabinoside, is a chemotherapy drug and is also known by its brand name, Ara C.

It is a treatment for:

- acute leukaemias (cancers of the blood)
- some lymphomas (cancers of the lymph glands)
- For some types of lymphoma you have cytarabine injected into the fluid around the spinal cord (intrathecally).

How it works

This drug is a type of chemotherapy drug called an anti-metabolite. Anti metabolites are similar to normal body molecules but they are slightly different in structure. They kill cancer cells by stopping them making and repairing DNA that they need to grow and multiply.

How you have it

You have cytarabine as an injection into your bloodstream (intravenously) or by injection just under the skin (subcutaneously).

Drugs into your bloodstream

You have the treatment through a drip into your arm or hand. A nurse puts a small tube (a cannula) into one of your veins and connects the drip to it. You might need a central line. This is a long plastic tube that gives the drugs into a large vein, either in your chest or through a vein in your arm. It stays in while you're having treatment, which may be for a few months.

Subcutaneous injection

You usually have injections under the skin (subcutaneous injection) into the stomach or thigh. You might have stinging or a dull ache for a short time after this type of injection. The skin in the area may go red and itchy for a while.

When you have it

Having cytarabine through a drip can take from 10 minutes to 2 hours, depending on the dose you have. You may have it every day for 10 days. Or you may have it for 5 days and then have a rest of 2 to 9 days before repeating the treatment.

Tests

You have blood tests before and during your treatment. They check your levels of blood cells and other substances in the blood. They also check how well your liver and kidneys are working.

Other medicines, foods and drink

Cancer drugs can interact with some other medicines and herbal products. Tell your doctor or pharmacist about any medicines you are taking. This includes vitamins, herbal supplements and over the counter remedies.

Pregnancy and contraception

This drug may harm a baby developing in the womb. It is important not to become pregnant or father a child while you are having treatment with this drug and for at least 6 months afterwards. Talk to your doctor or nurse about effective contraception before starting treatment.

Loss of fertility

It is not known whether this treatment affects fertility in people. Talk to your doctor before starting treatment if you think you may want to have a baby in the future.

Breastfeeding

Don't breastfeed during this treatment because the drug may come through into your breast milk.

Treatment for other conditions

Always tell other doctors, nurses, pharmacists or dentists that you're having this treatment if you need treatment for anything else, including teeth problems.

Immunisations

Don't have immunisations with live vaccines while you're having treatment and for up to 12 months afterwards. The length of time depends on the treatment you are having. Ask your doctor or pharmacist how long you should avoid live vaccinations.

In the UK, live vaccines include rubella, mumps, measles, BCG, yellow fever and the shingles vaccine (Zostavax).

You can:

- ☐ have other vaccines, but they might not give you as much protection as usual
- ☐ have the flu vaccine (as an injection)
- ☐ be in contact with other people who have had live vaccines as injections
- ☐ Avoid close contact with people who have recently had live vaccines taken by mouth (oral vaccines) such as oral polio or the typhoid vaccine.

This also includes the rotavirus vaccine given to babies. The virus is in the baby's poo for up to 2 weeks and could make you ill. So avoid changing their nappies for 2 weeks after their vaccination if possible. Or wear disposable gloves and wash your hands well afterwards. You should also avoid close contact with children who have had the flu vaccine nasal spray if your immune system is severely weakened.

Daunorubicin

Daunorubicin is a chemotherapy drug, it is used to treat acute leukaemias.

How daunorubicin works

Daunorubicin is a type of chemotherapy called an anti-tumour antibiotic. It blocks an enzyme called topoisomerase 2, so the cancer cell's DNA gets tangled up and the cell can't split into 2 new cells.

How you have daunorubicin

You have daunorubicin into your bloodstream. It is a red liquid.

Into your bloodstream

You have the treatment through a drip into your arm or hand. A nurse puts a small tube (a cannula) into one of your veins and connects the drip to it. You might need a central line. This is a long plastic tube that gives the drugs into a large vein, either in your chest or through a vein in your arm. It stays in while you're having treatment, which may be for a few months.

Central lines

You have the drug injected into a fast running drip connected to your cannula or central line over about 10 minutes.

Daunorubicin

You usually have daunorubicin chemotherapy as a course of several cycles of treatment. How often and when you have it depends on which type of leukaemia you have.

Tests

You have blood tests before and during your treatment. They check your levels of blood cells and other substances in the blood. They also check how well your liver and kidneys are working.

Side effects

We haven't listed all the side effects. It's very unlikely that you will have all of these side effects, but you might have some of them at the same time. How often and how severe the side effects are can vary from person to person. They also depend on what other treatments you're having. For example, your side effects could be worse if you're also having other drugs or radiotherapy.

When to contact your team

Your doctor, nurse or pharmacist will go through the possible side effects. They will monitor you closely during treatment and check how you are at your appointments. Contact your advice line as soon as possible if:

- ☐ you have severe side effects
- ☐ your side effects aren't getting any better
- ☐ your side effects are getting worse
- ☐ Early treatment can help manage side effects better.

Contact your doctor or nurse immediately if you have signs of infection, including a temperature above 37.5C or below 36C.

Possible side effects

You might have one or more of these side effects:

- ☐ increased risk of getting an infection
- ☐ breathlessness and looking pale
- ☐ bruising, bleeding gums or nosebleeds

- tiredness and weakness (fatigue)
- feeling or being sick
- hair loss
- sore mouth
- red or pink urine for a few days after treatment
- inflammation of mucous membranes, such as inside the mouth, nose, vagina or back passage (rectum)
- allergic reaction
- inflammation, pain and swelling at the drip site
- high temperature (fever) and chills
- tummy (abdominal) pain
- periods stopping
- dehydration
- heart damage
- severe infection (sepsis)

Coping with side effects

What else do I need to know?

Other medicines, foods and drink

Cancer drugs can interact with some other medicines and herbal products. Tell your doctor or pharmacist about any medicines you are taking. This includes vitamins, herbal supplements and over the counter remedies.

Pregnancy and contraception

This drug can harm a baby developing in the womb. You should avoid becoming pregnant, or fathering a child during treatment, and for 6 months after treatment. Talk to your team about reliable contraception before starting treatment.

Fertility

You may not be able to become pregnant or father a child after treatment with this drug. Talk to your doctor before starting treatment if you think you may want to have a baby in the future. Men may be able to store sperm before starting treatment. Women may be able to store eggs or ovarian tissue but this is rare.

Breastfeeding

Don't breastfeed during this treatment because the drug may come through into your breast milk.

Treatment for other conditions

Always tell other doctors, nurses, pharmacists or dentists that you're having this treatment if you need treatment for anything else, including teeth problems.

Immunisations

Don't have immunisations with live vaccines while you're having treatment and for up to 12 months afterwards. The length of time depends on the treatment you are having. Ask your doctor or pharmacist how long you should avoid live vaccinations. In the UK, live vaccines include rubella, mumps, measles, BCG, yellow fever and the shingles vaccine (Zostavax).

You can:

- have other vaccines, but they might not give you as much protection as usual
- have the flu vaccine (as an injection)
- be in contact with other people who have had live vaccines as injections
- Avoid close contact with people who have recently had live vaccines taken by mouth (oral vaccines) such as oral polio or the typhoid vaccine.

This also includes the rotavirus vaccine given to babies. The virus is in the baby's poo for up to 2 weeks and could make you ill. So avoid changing their nappies for 2 weeks after their vaccination if possible. Or wear disposable gloves and wash your hands well afterwards. You should also avoid close contact with children who have had the flu vaccine nasal spray if your immune system is severely weakened.

Doxorubicin (Adriamycin)

Find out what doxorubicin is, how you have it and other important information about having doxorubicin. Doxorubicin is a chemotherapy drug and is also known by its brand name Adriamycin.

It is a treatment for many different types of cancer.

How doxorubicin works

Doxorubicin is a type of chemotherapy drug called an anthracycline. It slows or stops the growth of cancer cells by blocking an enzyme called topo isomerase 2. Cancer cells need this enzyme to divide and grow. You might have doxorubicin in combination with other chemotherapy drugs.

How you have doxorubicin

You have doxorubicin into your bloodstream.

Drugs into your bloodstream

You have the treatment through a drip into your arm or hand. A nurse puts a small tube (a cannula) into one of your veins and connects the drip to it. You might need a central line. This is a long plastic tube that gives the drugs into a large vein, either in your chest or through a vein in your arm. It stays in while you're having treatment, which may be for a few months.

Central lines

Into the bladder

Sometimes, doxorubicin may be given directly into the bladder to treat cancer of the bladder lining. This is called intravesical chemotherapy and the side effects are different to doxorubicin given into a vein.

When you have it

You usually have this type of chemotherapy as a course of several cycles of treatment. The number of cycles you have depends on your treatment plan.

Tests

You have blood tests before and during your treatment. They check your levels of blood cells and other substances in the blood. They also check how well your liver and kidneys are working.

Other medicines, foods and drink

Cancer drugs can interact with some other medicines and herbal products. Tell your doctor or pharmacist about any medicines you are taking. This includes vitamins, herbal supplements and over the counter remedies.

Pregnancy and contraception

This drug may harm a baby developing in the womb. It is important not to become pregnant or father a child while you are having treatment with this drug and for at least 6 months afterwards. Talk to your doctor or nurse about effective contraception before starting treatment.

Fertility

You may not be able to become pregnant or father a child after treatment with this drug. Talk to your doctor before starting treatment if you think you may want to have a baby in the future. Men may be able to store sperm before starting treatment. Women may be able to store eggs or ovarian tissue but this is rare.

Breastfeeding

Don't breastfeed during this treatment because the drug may come through into your breast milk.

Treatment for other conditions

Always tell other doctors, nurses, pharmacists or dentists that you're having this treatment if you need treatment for anything else, including teeth problems.

If you have had radiotherapy

Tell your doctor if you have had radiotherapy treatment to your chest that might have been near to or involving your heart. This could increase the risk of heart damage from doxorubicin and your doctor will need to take this into account.

Immunisations

Don't have immunisations with live vaccines while you're having treatment and for up to 12 months afterwards. The length of time depends on the treatment you are having. Ask your doctor or pharmacist how long you should avoid live vaccinations. In the UK, live vaccines include rubella, mumps, measles, BCG, yellow fever and the shingles vaccine (Zostavax).

You can:

- have other vaccines, but they might not give you as much protection as usual
- have the flu vaccine (as an injection)

- be in contact with other people who have had live vaccines as injections
- Avoid close contact with people who have recently had live vaccines taken by mouth (oral vaccines) such as oral polio or the typhoid vaccine.

This also includes the rotavirus vaccine given to babies. The virus is in the baby's poo for up to 2 weeks and could make you ill. So avoid changing their nappies for 2 weeks after their vaccination if possible. Or wear disposable gloves and wash your hands well afterwards.

You should also avoid close contact with children who have had the flu vaccine nasal spray if your immune system is severely weakened.

Etoposide (Eposin, Etopophos, Vepesid)

Etoposide is a chemotherapy drug and is also known by its brand name, Eposin, Etopophos or Vepesid.

It is a treatment for several different types of cancer.

How it works

DNA is the genetic code that is in the nucleus of all animal and plant cells. It controls everything the cell does.

Etoposide works by blocking an enzyme (called topoisomerase 2) which is necessary for cancer cells to divide and so grow into 2 new cells. If this enzyme is blocked, the cell's DNA gets tangled up and the cell can't divide.

How you have it

You can have etoposide into your bloodstream (Eposin or Etopophos).

Or you can have etoposide as capsules (Vepesid). You have the capsules on an empty stomach.

Drugs into your bloodstream

You have the treatment through a drip into your arm or hand. A nurse puts a small tube (a cannula) into one of your veins and connects the drip to it. You might need a central line. This is a long plastic tube that gives the drugs into a large vein, either in your chest or through a vein in your arm. It stays in while you're having treatment, which may be for a few months.

Taking capsules

You must take your capsules according to the instructions your doctor or pharmacist gives you.

Whether you have a full or empty stomach can affect how much of a drug gets into your bloodstream.

☐ You should take the right dose, not more or less.

☐ When you have etoposide

You take the capsules each day, usually for 5 consecutive days every 3 weeks. If you have the drug into your bloodstream you usually have it as a course of several cycles of treatment.

Tests

You have blood tests before and during your treatment. They check your levels of blood cells and other substances in the blood. They also check how well your liver and kidneys are working.

Other medicines, foods and drink

Cancer drugs can interact with some other medicines and herbal products. Tell your doctor or pharmacist about any medicines you are taking. This includes vitamins, herbal supplements and over the counter remedies.

Pregnancy and contraception

This drug may harm a baby developing in the womb. It is important not to become pregnant or father a child while you are having treatment with this drug and for at least 6 months afterwards. Talk to your doctor or nurse about effective contraception before starting treatment.

Breastfeeding

Don't breastfeed during this treatment because the drug may come through into your breast milk.

Loss of fertility

☐ This treatment might stop you being able to father a child.

☐ Talk to your doctor before starting treatment if you think you may want to have a baby in the future.

You may be able to store sperm before starting treatment.

Usually, fertility returns to normal after a few months or sometimes years. You can have sperm counts to check your fertility when your treatment is over. Ask your doctor about it.

Treatment for other conditions

Always tell other doctors, nurses, pharmacists or dentists that you're having this treatment if you need treatment for anything else, including teeth problems.

Immunisations

Don't have immunisations with live vaccines while you're having treatment and for up to 12 months afterwards. The length of time depends on the treatment you are having. Ask your doctor or pharmacist how long you should avoid live vaccinations.

In the UK, live vaccines include rubella, mumps, measles, BCG, yellow fever and the shingles vaccine (Zostavax).

You can:

- ☐ have other vaccines, but they might not give you as much protection as usual
- ☐ have the flu vaccine (as an injection)
- ☐ be in contact with other people who have had live vaccines as injections
- ☐ Avoid close contact with people who have recently had live vaccines taken by mouth (oral vaccines) such

as oral polio or the typhoid vaccine.

This also includes the rotavirus vaccine given to babies. The virus is in the baby's poo for up to 2 weeks and could make you ill. So avoid changing their nappies for 2 weeks after their vaccination if possible. Or wear disposable gloves and wash your hands well afterwards. You should also avoid close contact with children who have had the flu vaccine nasal spray if your immune system is severely weakened.

Mercaptopurine (Xaluprine)

Mercaptopurine is also called Xaluprine. It is a chemotherapy drug used to treat some types of leukaemia.

How it works

Mercaptopurine is one of a group of chemotherapy drugs known as anti-metabolites. These drugs stop cells making and repairing DNA. Cancer cells need to make and repair DNA so that they can grow and multiply.

How you have it

Mercaptopurine comes as pale yellow tablets and as a pink to brown liquid (oral suspension). The liquid medicine is called Xaluprine.

Taking mercaptopurine tablets

You swallow the tablets whole with lots of water. You can take them with food, or on an empty stomach. You should take the tablets at the same time each day. You should not take them at the same time as milk or dairy products. You can take them:

1 hour before milk or dairy products

2 hours after milk or dairy products

If you need to break them in half, wash your hands afterwards and make sure that you don't breathe in any of the powder released by the tablet.

Taking mercaptopurine liquid

Your nurse or pharmacist will show you how to measure the dose of liquid mercaptopurine (Xaluprine) using a syringe. You need to wear disposable gloves while doing this so that the drug doesn't contact your skin. You take Xaluprine in the evening, with food or on an empty stomach. But whichever you choose, you should do the same thing each day. You should drink some water after taking the liquid. Milk and dairy products can make this drug less effective so you should take Xaluprine at least 1 hour before or 2 hours after milk or dairy products.

If you take too much mercaptopurine

If you accidentally take more mercaptopurine than you should you might feel sick, be sick or have diarrhoea. Tell your doctor or go to a hospital straight away. Take the medicine pack with you.

- If you forget to take mercaptopurine
- Don't take a double dose to make up for the dose that you forgot. Tell your doctor or nurse.

Taking your tablets or capsules

You must take tablets and capsules according to the instructions your doctor or pharmacist gives you.

- ☐ You should take the right dose, not more or less.
- ☐ Talk to your specialist or advice line before you stop taking a cancer drug.

When you have it

You usually have mercaptopurine as a course of several cycles of treatment. The treatment plan for mercaptopurine depends on which type of cancer you have.

Tests

You have blood tests before and during your treatment. They check your levels of blood cells and other substances in the blood. They also check how well your liver and kidneys are working.

Side effects

We haven't listed all the side effects. It's very unlikely that you will have all of these side effects, but you might have some of them at the same time. How often and how severe the side effects are can vary from person to person. They also depend on what other treatments you're having. For example, your side effects could be worse if you're also having other drugs or radiotherapy.

When to contact your team

Your doctor, nurse or pharmacist will go through the

possible side effects. They will monitor you closely during treatment and check how you are at your appointments. Contact your advice line as soon as possible if:

- you have severe side effects
- your side effects aren't getting any better
- your side effects are getting worse
- Early treatment can help manage side effects better.

Contact your doctor or nurse immediately if you have signs of infection, including a temperature above 37.5C or below 36C.

Common side effects

These effects happen in more than 1 in 10 people (10%). They include:

Increased risk of getting an infection

Increased risk of getting an infection is due to a drop in white blood cells. Symptoms include a change in temperature, aching muscles, headaches, feeling cold and shivery and generally unwell. You might have other symptoms depending on where the infection is. Infections can sometimes be life threatening. You should contact your advice line urgently if you think you have an infection.

Bruising, bleeding gums or nosebleeds

This is due to a drop in the number of platelets in your blood. These blood cells help the blood to clot when we cut ourselves. You may have nosebleeds or bleeding gums after brushing your teeth. Or you may have lots of tiny red spots or bruises on your arms or legs (known as petechia).

Occasional side effects

These effects happen in more than 1 in 100 people (1%). You might have one or more of them. They include:

- ☐ diarrhoea
- ☐ feeling or being sick
- ☐ breathlessness and looking pale (due to low red blood cell counts) and tiredness
- ☐ sore mouth
- ☐ changes to how your liver works
- ☐ blocked bile ducts

Rare side effects

These effects happen in fewer than 1 in 100 people (1%). You might have one or more of them. They include:

- ☐ loss of appetite
- ☐ skin changes (such as rash)
- ☐ inflammation of the pancreas
- ☐ aching muscles

Other medicines, foods and drink

Cancer drugs can interact with some other medicines and herbal products. Tell your doctor or pharmacist about any medicines you are taking. This includes vitamins, herbal supplements and over the counter remedies.

Pregnancy and contraception

This drug may harm a baby developing in the womb. It is important not to become pregnant or father a child while you are having treatment with this drug and for at least 3 months afterwards. Talk to your doctor or nurse about effective contraception before starting treatment.

Fertility

You may not be able to become pregnant or father a child after treatment with this drug. Talk to your doctor before starting treatment if you think you may want to have a baby in the future. Men may be able to store sperm before starting treatment. Women may be able to store eggs or ovarian tissue but this is rare.

Breastfeeding

Don't breastfeed during this treatment because the drug may come through into your breast milk.

Treatment for other conditions

Always tell other doctors, nurses, pharmacists or dentists that you're having this treatment if you need treatment for anything else, including teeth problems.

Lactose and mercaptopurine

This drug contains lactose (milk sugar). If you have an intolerance to lactose, contact your doctor before taking this medicine.

Immunisations

Don't have immunisations with live vaccines while you're having treatment and for up to 12 months afterwards. The length of time depends on the treatment you are having. Ask your doctor or pharmacist how long you should avoid live vaccinations. In the UK, live vaccines include rubella, mumps, measles, BCG, yellow fever and the shingles vaccine (Zostavax).

You can:

- have other vaccines, but they might not give you as much protection as usual
- have the flu vaccine (as an injection)
- be in contact with other people who have had live vaccines as injections
- Avoid close contact with people who have recently had live vaccines taken by mouth (oral vaccines) such as oral polio or the typhoid vaccine.

This also includes the rotavirus vaccine given to babies. The virus is in the baby's poo for up to 2 weeks and could make you ill. So avoid changing their nappies for 2 weeks after their vaccination if possible. Or wear disposable gloves and wash your hands well afterwards. You should also avoid close contact with children who have had the flu vaccine nasal spray if your immune system is severely weakened.

Mercaptopurine (Xaluprine)

Mercaptopurine is also called Xaluprine. It is a chemotherapy drug used to treat some types of leukaemia.

How it works

Mercaptopurine is one of a group of chemotherapy drugs known as anti-metabolites. These drugs stop cells making and repairing DNA. Cancer cells need to make and repair DNA so that they can grow and multiply.

How you have it

Mercaptopurine comes as pale yellow tablets and as a pink to brown liquid (oral suspension). The liquid medicine is called Xaluprine.

Taking mercaptopurine tablets

You swallow the tablets whole with lots of water. You can take them with food, or on an empty stomach. You should take the tablets at the same time each day. You should not take them at the same time as milk or dairy products. You can take them:

- 1 hour before milk or dairy products
- 2 hours after milk or dairy products
- If you need to break them in half, wash your hands afterwards and make sure that you don't breathe in any of the powder released by the tablet.

Taking mercaptopurine liquid

Your nurse or pharmacist will show you how to measure the dose of liquid mercaptopurine (Xaluprine) using a syringe. You need to wear disposable gloves while doing this so that the drug doesn't contact your skin. You take Xaluprine in the evening, with food or on an empty stomach. But whichever you choose, you should do the same thing each day. You should drink some water after taking the liquid. Milk and dairy products can make this drug less effective so you should take Xaluprine at least 1 hour before or 2 hours after milk or dairy products.

If you take too much mercaptopurine

If you accidentally take more mercaptopurine than you should you might feel sick, be sick or have diarrhoea. Tell your doctor or go to a hospital straight away. Take the medicine pack with you.

If you forget to take mercaptopurine

Don't take a double dose to make up for the dose that you forgot. Tell your doctor or nurse.

Taking your tablets or capsules

You must take tablets and capsules according to the instructions your doctor or pharmacist gives you. You should take the right dose, not more or less. Talk to your specialist or advice line before you stop taking a cancer drug.

When you have it

You usually have mercaptopurine as a course of several cycles of treatment. The treatment plan for mercaptopurine depends on which type of cancer you have.

Tests

You have blood tests before and during your treatment. They check your levels of blood cells and other substances in the blood. They also check how well your liver and kidneys are working.

Side effects

We haven't listed all the side effects. It's very unlikely that you will have all of these side effects, but you might have some of them at the same time. How often and how severe the side effects are can vary from person to person. They also depend on what other treatments you're having. For example, your side effects could be worse if you're also having other drugs or radiotherapy.

When to contact your team

Your doctor, nurse or pharmacist will go through the possible side effects. They will monitor you closely during treatment and check how you are at your appointments. Contact your advice line as soon as possible if:

- you have severe side effects
- your side effects aren't getting any better
- your side effects are getting worse
- Early treatment can help manage side effects better.

Contact your doctor or nurse immediately if you have signs of infection, including a temperature above 37.5C or below 36C.

Common side effects

These effects happen in more than 1 in 10 people (10%). They include:

Increased risk of getting an infection

Increased risk of getting an infection is due to a drop in white blood cells. Symptoms include a change in temperature, aching muscles, headaches, feeling cold and shivery and generally unwell. You might have other symptoms depending on where the infection is. Infections can sometimes be life threatening. You should contact your advice line urgently if you think you have an infection. This is due to a drop in the number of platelets in your blood. These blood cells help the blood to clot when we cut ourselves. You may have nosebleeds or bleeding gums after brushing your teeth. Or you may have lots of tiny red spots or bruises on your arms or legs (known as petechia).

Occasional side effects

These effects happen in more than 1 in 100 people (1%). You might have one or more of them. They include:

- diarrhoea
- feeling or being sick
- breathlessness and looking pale (due to low red blood cell counts) and tiredness
- sore mouth
- changes to how your liver works
- blocked bile ducts

Rare side effects

These effects happen in fewer than 1 in 100 people (1%). You might have one or more of them. They include:

- loss of appetite
- skin changes (such as rash)
- inflammation of the pancreas
- aching muscles

What else do I need to know?

Other medicines, foods and drink

Cancer drugs can interact with some other medicines and herbal products. Tell your doctor or pharmacist about any medicines you are taking. This includes vitamins, herbal supplements and over the counter remedies.

Pregnancy and contraception

This drug may harm a baby developing in the womb. It is important not to become pregnant or father a child while you are having treatment with this drug and for at least 3 months afterwards. Talk to your doctor or nurse about effective contraception before starting treatment.

Fertility

You may not be able to become pregnant or father a child after treatment with this drug. Talk to your doctor before starting treatment if you think you may want to have a baby in the future. Men may be able to store sperm before starting treatment. Women may be able to store eggs or ovarian tissue but this is rare.

Breastfeeding

Don't breastfeed during this treatment because the drug may come through into your breast milk.

Treatment for other conditions

Always tell other doctors, nurses, pharmacists or dentists that you're having this treatment if you need treatment for anything else, including teeth problems.

Lactose and mercaptopurine

This drug contains lactose (milk sugar). If you have an intolerance to lactose, contact your doctor before taking this medicine.

Immunisations

Don't have immunisations with live vaccines while you're having treatment and for up to 12 months afterwards. The length of time depends on the treatment you are having. Ask your doctor or pharmacist how long you should avoid live vaccinations. In the UK, live vaccines include rubella, mumps, measles, BCG, yellow fever and the shingles vaccine (Zostavax).

You can:

- have other vaccines, but they might not give you as much protection as usual
- have the flu vaccine (as an injection)

- be in contact with other people who have had live vaccines as injections
- Avoid close contact with people who have recently had live vaccines taken by mouth (oral vaccines) such as oral polio or the typhoid vaccine.

This also includes the rotavirus vaccine given to babies. The virus is in the baby's poo for up to 2 weeks and could make you ill. So avoid changing their nappies for 2 weeks after their vaccination if possible. Or wear disposable gloves and wash your hands well afterwards. You should also avoid close contact with children who have had the flu vaccine nasal spray if your immune system is severely weakened.

Methotrexate

Methotrexate is a type of chemotherapy. It's a treatment for a number of different types of cancer.

How methotrexate works

Methotrexate is one of a group of chemotherapy drugs called anti metabolites. These stop cells making and repairing DNA. Cancer cells need to make and repair DNA so that they can grow and multiply. Methotrexate stops the cells working properly. Methotrexate also stops some normal cells working properly, causing side effects. You might have another drug called folinic acid after methotrexate. It helps normal cells recover and reduces side effects.

How you have methotrexate

How you have methotrexate depends on what type of cancer you have. You can have it as:

- an injection into your bloodstream (intravenous)
- a tablet or a liquid you can drink (solution)
- an injection into your muscle
- an injection into your spinal fluid (intrathecal injection)
- Into your bloodstream

You might have the treatment through a drip into your arm. Your nurse puts a small tube (a cannula) into one of your veins and connects the drip to it.Or you might need a central line. This is a long plastic tube that gives the drugs into a large vein, either in your chest or through a vein in your arm. It stays in the whole time you are having treatment.

Central lines

Taking your tablets or liquid

You must take tablets and liquid according to the instructions your doctor or pharmacist gives you.

You should take the right dose, not more or less.

Never stop taking a cancer drug without talking to your specialist first.

Injection into your muscle (intramuscular)

- You have the injection into a muscle, usually into your buttock or upper thigh.

- Injection into your spinal fluid

Your doctor injects the drug into the fluid around your spinal cord during a lumbar puncture. The side effects may be less with this way of having methotrexate but it can cause:

- a headache
- high temperature (fever)
- stiff neck
- back or shoulder pain
- sleepiness
- temporary shaking (tremor)
- irritability and confusion
- feeling or being sick
- difficult or unclear speech
- fits (seizures)
- swelling in the brain

When you have methotrexate

You usually have it as a course of several cycles of treatment. Each cycle varies depending on what type of cancer you have. Your doctor or nurse will tell you more about this.

Tests

You have blood tests before and during your treatment. They check your levels of blood cells and other substances in the blood. They also check how well your liver and kidneys are working.

Side effects

Side effects of treatment will depend on the amount you have (the dose) and how you have the drug. We haven't listed all the side effects. Your doctor or nurse will talk to you about the possible side effects. Tell them if you notice anything unusual or different during and after treatment.

When to contact your team

Your doctor and nurse will monitor you closely for any side effects. Let them know as soon as possible if:

- you have severe side effects
- your side effects aren't getting any better
- your side effects are getting worse
- Early treatment can help manage side effects better.

Contact your doctor or nurse immediately if you have signs of infection, including a temperature above 37.5C.

Common side effects

Each of these side effects happens in more than 1 and 10 people (10%). You might have one or more of them. They include:

Increased risk of infection

Increased risk of getting an infection is due to a drop in white blood cells. Symptoms include a change in temperature, aching muscles, headaches, feeling cold and shivery and generally unwell. You might have other symptoms depending on where the infection is. Infections can sometimes be life threatening. You should contact your advice line urgently if you think you have an infection.

Bruising, bleeding gums and nosebleeds

This is due to a drop in the number of platelets in your blood. These blood cells help the blood to clot when we cut ourselves. You may have nosebleeds or bleeding gums after brushing your teeth. Or you may have lots of tiny red spots or bruises on your arms or legs (known as petechia).

Mouth sores and ulcers

Mouth sores and ulcers can be painful. Keep your mouth and teeth clean; drink plenty of fluids; avoid acidic foods such as oranges, lemons and grapefruits; chew gum to keep the mouth moist and tell your doctor or nurse if you have ulcers.

Liver changes

You might have liver changes that are usually mild and unlikely to cause symptoms. They usually go back to normal when treatment finishes. You have regular blood tests to check for any changes in the way your liver is working.

Indigestion or heartburn

Contact your doctor or pharmacist if you have indigestion or heartburn. They can prescribe medicines to help.

Tummy (abdominal) pain

Tell your treatment team if you have this. They can check the cause and give you medicine to help.

Feeling or being sick

Feeling or being sick is usually well controlled with anti-sickness medicines. Avoiding fatty or fried foods, eating small meals and snacks, drinking plenty of water, and relaxation techniques, can all help.

Loss of appetite

You might not feel like eating and may lose weight. It is important to eat as much as you can. Eating several small meals and snacks throughout the day can be easier to manage. You can talk to a dietitian if you are concerned about your appetite or weight loss.

Kidney changes

You might have some changes in the way your kidneys work. You'll have regular blood tests to check how well they are working.

Occasional side effects

Each of these effects happens in more than 1 in 100 people (1%). You might have one or more of them. They include:

- breathlessness and looking pale due to a drop in red blood cells (anaemia)
- tiredness (fatigue)

- headaches
- drowsiness
- dizziness
- diarrhoea
- skin changes such as a rash, itching or reddening of the skin
- thickening and scarring of the lung tissue causing a cough and shortness of breath
- hair loss - usually with higher doses of methotrexate, for example lymphoma

Rare side effects

Each of these effects happens in fewer than 1 in 100 people (less than 1%). You might have one or more of them. They include:

- an allergic reaction that can cause a rash, shortness of breath, redness or swelling of the face and dizziness
- confusion
- depression
- high blood sugar levels (diabetes)
- your skin and eyes being very sensitive to sunlight
- muscle and joint pain
- weakening of the bones (osteoporosis)
- ulcers and swelling (inflammation) of the stomach and bowel, bladder or vagina
- fits (seizures)

- weakness on one side of your body

a severe skin reaction that may start as tender red patches which leads to peeling or blistering of the skin. You might also feel feverish and your eyes may be more sensitive to light. This is serious and could be life threatening a second cancer called lymphoma.

Other medicines, foods and drink

Cancer drugs can interact with some other medicines and herbal products. Tell your doctor or pharmacist about any medicines you are taking. This includes vitamins, herbal supplements and over the counter remedies. It is important to drink plenty during treatment for methotrexate. If you become dehydrated you may increase the side effects of the drug.

Avoid drinking alcohol while having methotrexate.

Pregnancy and contraception

This treatment might harm a baby developing in the womb. It is important not to become pregnant or father a child while you're having treatment and for up to 12 months afterwards. Talk to your doctor or nurse about effective contraception before starting treatment.

Breastfeeding

Don't breastfeed during this treatment because the drug may come through into your breast milk.

Treatment for other conditions

Always tell other doctors, nurses, pharmacists or dentists that you're having this treatment if you need treatment for anything else, including teeth problems.

Fertility

You may not be able to become pregnant or father a child after treatment with this drug. Talk to your doctor before starting treatment if you think you may want to have a baby in the future. Men may be able to store sperm before starting treatment. Women may be able to store eggs or ovarian tissue but this is rare.

Driving and use of machinery

This drug can cause tiredness and dizziness. Don't drive or operate heavy machinery if you have these symptoms.

Immunisations

Don't have immunisations with live vaccines while you're having treatment and for up to 12 months afterwards. The length of time depends on the treatment you are having. Ask your doctor or pharmacist how long you should avoid live vaccinations. In the UK, live vaccines include rubella, mumps, measles, BCG, yellow fever and the shingles vaccine (Zostavax).

You can:

- ☐ have other vaccines, but they might not give you as much protection as usual
- ☐ have the flu vaccine (as an injection)

- be in contact with other people who have had live vaccines as injections
- Avoid close contact with people who have recently had live vaccines taken by mouth (oral vaccines) such as oral polio or the typhoid vaccine.

This also includes the rotavirus vaccine given to babies. The virus is in the baby's poo for up to 2 weeks and could make you ill. So avoid changing their nappies for 2 weeks after their vaccination if possible. Or wear disposable gloves and wash your hands well afterwards. You should also avoid close contact with children who have had the flu vaccine nasal spray if your immune system is severely weakened.

Methotrexate

Methotrexate is a type of chemotherapy. It's a treatment for a number of different types of cancer.

How methotrexate works

Methotrexate is one of a group of chemotherapy drugs called anti metabolites. These stop cells making and repairing DNA. Cancer cells need to make and repair DNA so that they can grow and multiply. Methotrexate stops the cells working properly. Methotrexate also stops some normal cells working properly, causing side effects. You might have another drug called folinic acid after methotrexate. It helps normal cells recover and reduces side effects.

How you have methotrexate

How you have methotrexate depends on what type of cancer you have. You can have it as:

- an injection into your bloodstream (intravenous)
- a tablet or a liquid you can drink (solution)
- an injection into your muscle
- an injection into your spinal fluid (intrathecal injection)
- Into your bloodstream

You might have the treatment through a drip into your arm. Your nurse puts a small tube (a cannula) into one of your veins and connects the drip to it. Or you might need a central line. This is a long plastic tube that gives the drugs into a large vein, either in your chest or through a vein in your arm. It stays in the whole time you are having treatment.

Central lines

- Taking your tablets or liquid
- You must take tablets and liquid according to the instructions your doctor or pharmacist gives you.
- You should take the right dose, not more or less.
- Never stop taking a cancer drug without talking to your specialist first.
- Injection into your muscle (intramuscular)
- You have the injection into a muscle, usually into your buttock or upper thigh.
- Injection into your spinal fluid

Your doctor injects the drug into the fluid around your

spinal cord during a lumbar puncture. The side effects may be less with this way of having methotrexate but it can cause:

- a headache
- high temperature (fever)
- stiff neck
- back or shoulder pain
- sleepiness
- temporary shaking (tremor)
- irritability and confusion
- feeling or being sick
- difficult or unclear speech
- fits (seizures)
- swelling in the brain

When you have methotrexate

You usually have it as a course of several cycles of treatment. Each cycle varies depending on what type of cancer you have. Your doctor or nurse will tell you more about this.

Tests

You have blood tests before and during your treatment. They check your levels of blood cells and other substances in the blood. They also check how well your liver and kidneys are working.

Side effects

Side effects of treatment will depend on the amount you have (the dose) and how you have the drug.

We haven't listed all the side effects. Your doctor or nurse will talk to you about the possible side effects. Tell them if you notice anything unusual or different during and after treatment.

When to contact your team

Your doctor and nurse will monitor you closely for any side effects. Let them know as soon as possible if:

- you have severe side effects
- your side effects aren't getting any better
- your side effects are getting worse
- Early treatment can help manage side effects better.

Contact your doctor or nurse immediately if you have signs of infection, including a temperature above 37.5C.

Common side effects

Each of these side effects happens in more than 1 and 10 people (10%). You might have one or more of them. They include:

Increased risk of infection

Increased risk of getting an infection is due to a drop in white blood cells. Symptoms include a change in temperature, aching muscles, headaches, feeling cold and shivery and generally unwell. You might have other symptoms depending on where the infection is. Infections can sometimes be life threatening. You should contact your advice line urgently if you think you have an infection.

Bruising, bleeding gums and nosebleeds

This is due to a drop in the number of platelets in your blood. These blood cells help the blood to clot when we cut ourselves. You may have nosebleeds or bleeding gums after brushing your teeth. Or you may have lots of tiny red spots or bruises on your arms or legs (known as petechia).

Mouth sores and ulcers

Mouth sores and ulcers can be painful. Keep your mouth and teeth clean; drink plenty of fluids; avoid acidic foods such as oranges, lemons and grapefruits; chew gum to keep the mouth moist and tell your doctor or nurse if you have ulcers.

Liver changes

You might have liver changes that are usually mild and unlikely to cause symptoms. They usually go back to normal when treatment finishes. You have regular blood tests to check for any changes in the way your liver is working.

Indigestion or heartburn

Contact your doctor or pharmacist if you have indigestion or heartburn. They can prescribe medicines to help.

Tummy (abdominal) pain

Tell your treatment team if you have this. They can check the cause and give you medicine to help.

Feeling or being sick

Feeling or being sick is usually well controlled with anti-sickness medicines. Avoiding fatty or fried foods, eating small meals and snacks, drinking plenty of water, and relaxation techniques, can all help.

Loss of appetite

You might not feel like eating and may lose weight. It is important to eat as much as you can. Eating several small meals and snacks throughout the day can be easier to manage. You can talk to a dietitian if you are concerned about your appetite or weight loss.

Kidney changes

You might have some changes in the way your kidneys work. You'll have regular blood tests to check how well they are working.

Occasional side effects

Each of these effects happens in more than 1 in 100 people (1%). You might have one or more of them. They include:

- ☐ breathlessness and looking pale due to a drop in red blood cells (anaemia)
- ☐ tiredness (fatigue)

- headaches
- drowsiness
- dizziness
- diarrhoea
- skin changes such as a rash, itching or reddening of the skin
- thickening and scarring of the lung tissue causing a cough and shortness of breath
- hair loss - usually with higher doses of methotrexate, for example lymphoma

Rare side effects

Each of these effects happens in fewer than 1 in 100 people (less than 1%). You might have one or more of them. They include:

- an allergic reaction that can cause a rash, shortness of breath, redness or swelling of the face and dizziness
- confusion
- depression
- high blood sugar levels (diabetes)
- your skin and eyes being very sensitive to sunlight
- muscle and joint pain
- weakening of the bones (osteoporosis)
- ulcers and swelling (inflammation) of the stomach and bowel, bladder or vagina
- fits (seizures)

☐ weakness on one side of your body

a severe skin reaction that may start as tender red patches which leads to peeling or blistering of the skin. You might also feel feverish and your eyes may be more sensitive to light. This is serious and could be life threatening second cancer called lymphoma.

Other medicines, foods and drink

Cancer drugs can interact with some other medicines and herbal products. Tell your doctor or pharmacist about any medicines you are taking. This includes vitamins, herbal supplements and over the counter remedies. It is important to drink plenty during treatment for methotrexate. If you become dehydrated you may increase the side effects of the drug.

☐ Avoid drinking alcohol while having methotrexate.

☐ Pregnancy and contraception

This treatment might harm a baby developing in the womb. It is important not to become pregnant or father a child while you're having treatment and for up to 12 months afterwards. Talk to your doctor or nurse about effective contraception before starting treatment.

Breastfeeding

Don't breastfeed during this treatment because the drug may come through into your breast milk.

Treatment for other conditions

Always tell other doctors, nurses, pharmacists or dentists

that you're having this treatment if you need treatment for anything else, including teeth problems.

Fertility

You may not be able to become pregnant or father a child after treatment with this drug. Talk to your doctor before starting treatment if you think you may want to have a baby in the future. Men may be able to store sperm before starting treatment. Women may be able to store eggs or ovarian tissue but this is rare.

Driving and use of machinery

This drug can cause tiredness and dizziness. Don't drive or operate heavy machinery if you have these symptoms.

Immunisations

Don't have immunisations with live vaccines while you're having treatment and for up to 12 months afterwards. The length of time depends on the treatment you are having. Ask your doctor or pharmacist how long you should avoid live vaccinations. In the UK, live vaccines include rubella, mumps, measles, BCG, yellow fever and the shingles vaccine (Zostavax).

You can:

- have other vaccines, but they might not give you as much protection as usual
- have the flu vaccine (as an injection)
- be in contact with other people who have had live vaccines as injections

- Avoid close contact with people who have recently had live vaccines taken by mouth (oral vaccines) such as oral polio or the typhoid vaccine.

This also includes the rotavirus vaccine given to babies. The virus is in the baby's poo for up to 2 weeks and could make you ill. So avoid changing their nappies for 2 weeks after their vaccination if possible. Or wear disposable gloves and wash your hands well afterwards. You should also avoid close contact with children who have had the flu vaccine nasal spray if your immune system is severely weakened.

Nelarabine (Atriance)

Nelarabine is a chemotherapy drug and is also known by its brand name, Atriance.

It is a treatment for:

- a type of leukaemia called T cell acute lymphoblastic leukaemia
- a type of lymphoma called T cell lymphoblastic lymphoma
- Nelarabine is licensed but not yet approved for the whole of the UK.

You might have it if your leukaemia or lymphoma has come back after at least 2 other chemotherapy treatments.

How it works

Nelarabine is from a group of drugs known as antimetabolites.

Antimetabolites are similar to normal body molecules but they have a slightly different structure. They stop leukaemia and lymphoma cells making and repairing DNA so the cells can't grow and multiply.

How you have it

You have nelarabine as a drip (infusion) into your bloodstream (intravenously).

Drugs into your bloodstream

You have the treatment through a drip into your arm or hand. A nurse puts a small tube (a cannula) into one of your veins and connects the drip to it. You might need a central line. This is a long plastic tube that gives the drugs into a large vein, either in your chest or through a vein in your arm. It stays in while you're having treatment, which may be for a few months.

Central lines

When you have it

You usually have nelarabine as a course of several cycles of treatment. Each cycle of treatment lasts 21 days (3 weeks).

You have each treatment cycle in the following way:

Day 1

You have nelarabine as a drip into your bloodstream over 2 hours

Day 2

You have no treatment

Day 3

You have nelarabine as a drip into your bloodstream

Day 4

You have no treatment

Day 5

You have nelarabine as a drip into your bloodstream

Day 6 to 21

- You have no treatment
- Then you start the next treatment cycle.
- Nelarabine for children and young adults
- You usually have nelarabine infusion once a day for 5 days, if you are aged 21 or younger.
- It takes about an hour each time you have it. You have treatment every 3 weeks.
- Treatment to stop the build-up of uric acid
- As well as nelarabine, you might also have a drip to help stop the build-up of uric acid. Uric acid can build up in your body when cancer cells are broken down.

Tests

You have blood tests before and during your treatment. They check your levels of blood cells and other substances in the blood. They also check how well your liver and kidneys are working.

Other medicines, foods and drink

Cancer drugs can interact with some other medicines and herbal products. Tell your doctor or pharmacist about any medicines you are taking. This includes vitamins, herbal supplements and over the counter remedies.

Sodium and nelarabine

This drug contains sodium (salt). You might need to take account of this if you are on a controlled sodium diet. Tell your doctor if you are on a low salt diet.

Pregnancy and contraception

This drug may harm a baby developing in the womb. It is important not to become pregnant or father a child while you are having treatment with this drug and for at least 3 months afterwards. Talk to your doctor or nurse about effective contraception before starting treatment.

Fertility

It is not known whether this treatment affects fertility in people. Talk to your doctor before starting treatment if you think you may want to have a baby in the future.

Breastfeeding

Don't breastfeed during this treatment because the drug may come through into your breast milk.

Treatment for other conditions

Always tell other doctors, nurses, pharmacists or dentists that you're having this treatment if you need treatment for anything else, including teeth problems.

Immunisations

Don't have immunisations with live vaccines while you're having treatment and for up to 12 months afterwards. The length of time depends on the treatment you are having. Ask your doctor or pharmacist how long you should avoid live vaccinations. In the UK, live vaccines include rubella, mumps, measles, BCG, yellow fever and the shingles vaccine (Zostavax).

You can:

- have other vaccines, but they might not give you as much protection as usual
- have the flu vaccine (as an injection)
- be in contact with other people who have had live vaccines as injections

Avoid close contact with people who have recently had live vaccines taken by mouth (oral vaccines) such as oral polio or the typhoid vaccine. This also includes the rotavirus vaccine given to babies. The virus is in the baby's poo for up to 2 weeks and could make you ill. So avoid changing their nappies for 2 weeks after their vaccination if possible. Or wear disposable gloves and wash your hands well afterwards. You should also avoid close contact with children who have had the flu vaccine nasal spray if your immune system is severely weakened.

Tioguanine (thioguanine, 6-TG, 6-tioguanine)

Tioguanine is a chemotherapy drug and is also known as

thioguanine, 6-TG or 6-tioguanine.

It is a treatment for:

- [ ] acute myeloid leukaemia
- [ ] acute lymphoblastic leukaemia
- [ ] chronic myeloid leukaemia

How it works

Tioguanine is one of a group of chemotherapy drugs known as anti-metabolites. These drugs stop cells making and repairing DNA. Cancer cells need to make and repair DNA so that they can grow and multiply.

How you have it

You have tioguanine as tablets.

Take them on an empty stomach with plenty of water (for example, at least 1 hour before or 2 hours after meals). If you need to break your tablet in half, wash your hands straight afterwards. Be careful not to breathe in any powder that the tablet releases. If you accidentally take more tioguanine than you should tell your doctor straight away or go to a hospital. Take the medicine pack with you.

If you forget to take tioguanine tell your doctor. Don't take a double dose to make up for the missed dose.

Taking your tablets

- [ ] You must take tablets according to the instructions your doctor or pharmacist gives you.
- [ ] You should take the right dose, not more or less.

☐ Talk to your specialist or advice line before you stop taking a cancer drug.

When you have tioguanine

You usually have tioguanine chemotherapy as a course of several cycles of treatment. The treatment plan depends on which type of cancer you have.

Tests

You have blood tests before and during your treatment. They check your levels of blood cells and other substances in the blood. They also check how well your liver and kidneys are working.

Other medicines, foods and drink

Cancer drugs can interact with some other medicines and herbal products. Tell your doctor or pharmacist about any medicines you are taking. This includes vitamins, herbal supplements and over the counter remedies.

Pregnancy and contraception

This treatment might harm a baby developing in the womb. It is important not to become pregnant or father a child while you're having treatment and for a few months afterwards. Talk to your doctor or nurse about effective contraception before starting treatment.

Fertility

You may not be able to become pregnant or father a child

after treatment with this drug. Talk to your doctor before starting treatment if you think you may want to have a baby in the future. Men may be able to store sperm before starting treatment. Women may be able to store eggs or ovarian tissue but this is rare.

Breastfeeding

Don't breastfeed during this treatment because the drug may come through into your breast milk.

Treatment for other conditions

Always tell other doctors, nurses, pharmacists or dentists that you're having this treatment if you need treatment for anything else, including teeth problems.

Lesche-Nyhan syndrome

It is possible that tioguanine may not work for people who have Lesche-Nyhan syndrome. This syndrome is an inherited disorder in which people have very low levels of a protein needed to make tioguanine work.

TPMT (thiopurine methyltransferase)

Tioguanine may cause very severe side effects if you have a condition where your body produces too little of something called TPMT (thiopurine methyltransferase). Your doctor may do blood tests to check the levels before you start treatment.

Immunisations

Don't have immunisations with live vaccines while you're having treatment and for up to 12 months afterwards. The length of time depends on the treatment you are having. Ask your doctor or pharmacist how long you should avoid live vaccinations. In the UK, live vaccines include rubella, mumps, measles, BCG, yellow fever and the shingles vaccine (Zostavax).

You can:

- have other vaccines, but they might not give you as much protection as usual
- have the flu vaccine (as an injection)
- be in contact with other people who have had live vaccines as injections
- Avoid close contact with people who have recently had live vaccines taken by mouth (oral vaccines) such as oral polio or the typhoid vaccine.

This also includes the rotavirus vaccine given to babies. The virus is in the baby's poo for up to 2 weeks and could make you ill. So avoid changing their nappies for 2 weeks after their vaccination if possible. Or wear disposable gloves and wash your hands well afterwards. You should also avoid close contact with children who have had the flu vaccine nasal spray if your immune system is severely weakened.

Vincristine

Vincristine is a chemotherapy drug used to treat several different types of cancer.

How it works

- Vincristine is a chemotherapy drug that belongs to a group of drugs called vinca alkaloids.
- Vincristine works by stopping the cancer cells from separating into 2 new cells. So, it stops the growth of the cancer.

How you have it

You have vincristine into your bloodstream (intravenously).

Drugs into your bloodstream

You have the treatment through a drip into your arm or hand. A nurse puts a small tube (a cannula) into one of your veins and connects the drip to it. You might need a central line. This is a long plastic tube that gives the drugs into a large vein, either in your chest or through a vein in your arm. It stays in while you're having treatment, which may be for a few months.

Tests

You have blood tests before and during your treatment. They check your levels of blood cells and other substances in the blood. They also check how well your liver and kidneys are working.

Side effects

We haven't listed all the side effects. It's very unlikely that you will have all of these side effects, but you might have some of them at the same time. How often and how severe the side effects are can vary from person to person. They also depend on what other treatments you're having. For example, your side effects could be worse if you're also having other drugs or radiotherapy.

When to contact your team

Your doctor, nurse or pharmacist will go through the possible side effects. They will monitor you closely during treatment and check how you are at your appointments. Contact your advice line as soon as possible if:

☐ you have severe side effects

☐ your side effects aren't getting any better

☐ your side effects are getting worse

☐ Early treatment can help manage side effects better.

Contact your doctor or nurse immediately if you have signs of infection, including a temperature above 37.5C or below 36C.

You might have one or more of these side effects. They include:

☐ Increased risk of getting an infection

☐ Increased risk of getting an infection is due to a drop in white blood cells. Symptoms include a change in temperature, aching muscles, headaches, feeling cold and shivery and generally unwell. You might have other symptoms depending on where the infection is.

Infections can sometimes be life threatening. You should contact your advice line urgently if you think you have an infection.

Hair loss

You could lose all your hair. This includes your eyelashes, eyebrows, underarm, leg and sometimes pubic hair. Your hair will usually grow back once treatment has finished but it is likely to be softer. It may grow back a different colour or be curlier than before.

- Numbness or tingling in fingers or toes
- Numbness or tingling in fingers or toes is often temporary and can improve after you finish treatment. Talk to the team looking after you when you first notice this.

Tiredness and weakness (fatigue) during and after treatment

Tiredness and weakness (fatigue) can happen during and after treatment - doing gentle exercises each day can keep your energy up. Don't push yourself, rest when you start to feel tired and ask others for help.

Feeling or being sick

Feeling or being sick is usually well controlled with anti-sickness medicines. Avoiding fatty or fried foods, eating small meals and snacks, drinking plenty of water, and relaxation techniques, can all help.

Constipation

Constipation is easier to sort out if you treat it early. Drink plenty of fluids and eat as much fresh fruit and vegetables as you can. Try to take gentle exercise, such as walking. Tell your doctor or nurse if you are constipated for more than 3 days. They can prescribe a laxative.

Tummy (abdominal) pain

Tell your treatment team if you have this. They can check the cause and give you medicine to help.

- Periods stopping
- This might only be temporary.
- Changes to your eyesight
- Tell the team looking after you if you notice any changes or have pain.
- High temperature (fever) in children
- Your nurse will monitor this regularly.
- Difficulty passing urine

Let your doctor know if you are having this.

Muscle or bone pain

You might feel some pain from your muscles and joints. Speak to your doctor or nurse about what painkillers you can take to help with this.

Sore mouth and throat

It may be painful to swallow drinks or food. Painkillers and mouth washes can help to reduce the soreness and keep your mouth healthy.

Swelling and pain at the drip site

Tell your nurse straight away if you notice any signs of redness, swelling or leaking at your drip site.

Allergic reaction

A reaction may happen during the infusion, causing a skin rash, itching, swelling of the lips, face or throat, breathing difficulties, fever and chills. Your nurse will give you medicines beforehand to try to prevent a reaction. Tell your nurse or doctor immediately if at any time you feel unwell. They will slow or stop your drip for a while.

Taste changes

Taste changes may make you go off certain foods and drinks. You may also find that some foods taste different from usual or that you prefer to eat spicier foods. Your taste gradually goes back to normal a few weeks after your treatment finishes.

Hearing changes

You might have some hearing loss, especially with high pitched sounds. Tell your doctor or nurse if you notice any changes.

Loss of appetite and weight loss

You might not feel like eating and may lose weight. It is important to eat as much as you can. Eating several small meals and snacks throughout the day can be easier to manage. You can talk to a dietitian if you are concerned about your appetite or weight loss.

- ☐ Jaw pain
- ☐ Let your doctor know if you have this.
- ☐ Bowel not working
- ☐ Talk to your doctor about any changes to your bowel habits.

Skin rash

Skin problems include a skin rash, dry skin and itching. This usually goes back to normal when your treatment finishes. Your nurse will tell you what products you can use on your skin to help.

Headaches

Let your doctor or nurse know if you have headaches. They can give you painkillers. Don't drive or operate heavy machinery if you feel dizzy.

Diarrhoea

Contact your advice line if you have diarrhoea, such as if you've had 4 or more loose watery poos (stools) in 24 hours. Or if you can't drink to replace the lost fluid. Or if it carries on for more than 3 days. Your doctor may give you anti diarrhoea medicine to take home with you after treatment. Eat less fibre, avoid raw fruits, fruit juice, cereals and vegetables, and drink plenty to replace the fluid lost.

Other medicines, foods and drink

Cancer drugs can interact with some other medicines and herbal products. Tell your doctor or pharmacist about any medicines you are taking. This includes vitamins, herbal supplements and over the counter remedies.

Pregnancy and contraception

This treatment might harm a baby developing in the womb. It is important not to become pregnant or father a child while you are having treatment and for a few months afterwards. Talk to your doctor or nurse about effective contraception before starting treatment.

Fertility

You may not be able to become pregnant or father a child after treatment with this drug. Talk to your doctor before starting treatment if you think you may want to have a baby in the future. Men may be able to store sperm before starting treatment. Women may be able to store eggs or ovarian tissue but this is rare.

Breastfeeding

Don't breastfeed during this treatment because the drug may come through into your breast milk.

Treatment for other conditions

Always tell other doctors, nurses, pharmacists or dentists that you're having this treatment if you need treatment for anything else, including teeth problems.

Immunisations

Don't have immunisations with live vaccines while you're having treatment and for up to 12 months afterwards. The length of time depends on the treatment you are having. Ask your doctor or pharmacist how long you should avoid live vaccinations. In the UK, live vaccines include rubella, mumps, measles, BCG, yellow fever and the shingles vaccine (Zostavax).

You can:

- have other vaccines, but they might not give you as much protection as usual
- have the flu vaccine (as an injection)
- be in contact with other people who have had live vaccines as injections
- Avoid close contact with people who have recently had live vaccines taken by mouth (oral vaccines) such as oral polio or the typhoid vaccine.

This also includes the rotavirus vaccine given to babies. The virus is in the baby's poo for up to 2 weeks and could make you ill. So avoid changing their nappies for 2 weeks after their vaccination if possible. Or wear disposable gloves and wash your hands well afterwards. You should also avoid close contact with children who have had the flu vaccine nasal spray if your immune system is severely weakened.

Steroids

Steroids are naturally made by our bodies in small amounts. They help to control many functions. But steroids can also be made artificially and used as drugs to treat acute lymphoblastic leukaemia (ALL). Steroids used to treat ALL are usually a type called corticosteroids. These are man-made versions of the hormones produced by the adrenal glands just above the kidneys.

Corticosteroids include:

- prednisolone
- dexamethasone
- methylprednisolone

How you have steroids

You have steroids as tablets or liquid (if this is easier) to swallow. You take them after a meal or with milk as they can irritate your stomach. You can also have steroids as an injection into a muscle (intramuscular) or as an injection into a vein (intravenous).

Having an injection into a muscle or a vein

You must take the steroids according to the instructions your doctor or pharmacist gives you. You should take the right dose, not more or less. Never stop taking them without talking to your specialist first.

Taking medications safely

Side effects

Taking steroids as part of your treatment for ALL can cause side effects. These include:

- an increase in your appetite

- weight gain
- an increase in your energy levels
- difficulty sleeping
- indigestion or heartburn
- an increased risk of infection
- Fluid build up

Steroids can cause water retention if you take them for some time. You may notice some swelling in your hands, feet or eyelids and you may put on weight. This is due to extra fluid in your body. Let your doctor or nurse know if this happens to you.

Changes to blood sugar levels

You may need to go for a wee (pass urine) more often. And you may feel thirsty a lot of the time. This could be a sign that there are changes to your blood sugar levels. Your nurse checks your urine and blood for these changes. Some people are diagnosed with steroid induced diabetes whilst taking steroids. This doesn't mean you are a diabetic. Your sugar levels usually go back to normal after you stop taking the steroids. You learn how to test your urine for sugar at home or you bring urine samples to the hospital for testing. You might need to change your diet whilst taking the steroids. Your nurse will advise you.

- Mood changes
- Steroids can affect your mood. You might feel:
- anxious
- more emotional than usual

☐ low in mood and sad

☐ Tell your nurse or doctor if this is happening to you.

Rarely, steroids can cause a reaction called steroid induced psychosis. People can become excited, confused and imagine things that aren't real. This can be frightening, but it goes away when you stop taking the steroids.

Targeted cancer drugs and immunotherapy

Targeted cancer drugs work by targeting the differences in cancer cells that help them to grow and survive. Other drugs help the immune system to attack the cancer. They are called immunotherapies. These drugs are used for some types of ALL.

Targeted cancer drugs

The main targeted cancer drugs used for ALL are tyrosine kinase inhibitors or TKIs. They block tyrosine kinases, which are proteins cells use to signal to each other. Some of these signalling systems tell the cancer cells to grow and divide. So blocking the signals stops the cells from growing.

Doctors use TKIs to help treat a type of ALL called Philadelphia positive ALL (Ph+ ALL). About 20 to 30 out of every 100 people with ALL (about 20 to 30%) have this type. You most often have a TKI called imatinib (Glivec). You take it as a tablet. You usually have it with chemotherapy.

You might have a different TKI if the ALL comes back, such as:

- dasatinib (Sprycel)
- ponatinib (Iclusig)

Side effects

All treatments can cause side effects. While there are general side effects for a type of treatment, they vary for each individual drug. General side effects of these types of drugs include:

- fatigue (tiredness)
- diarrhoea
- skin changes such as a rash
- feeling or being sick

low blood cell counts – a drop in white blood cells mean you are at higher risk of picking up infections Tell your doctor or nurse if you have any side effects. They can usually give medicines to help control them.

Drugs that help the body's immune system (immunotherapy)

Doctors may use a type of immunotherapy called a monoclonal antibody to help treat pre B cell ALL. This is the most common type of ALL in adults. These drugs work by attaching to the leukaemia cells so that the immune system can find and destroy them.

You might have:

- blinatumomab (Blincyto)
- inotuzumab ozogamicin (Besponsa)

You have one of these drugs on its own to help treat ALL that has come back or is not responding to treatment. You have it through a drip into your bloodstream.

Side effects

The side effects depend on the drug you are having. Some of the common side effects include:

- flu-like symptoms including a high temperature, sore throat, shivering and muscle aches
- headaches and dizziness
- bleeding
- tummy (abdominal) pain
- diarrhoea or constipation
- feeling or being sick
- skin problems such as a rash

a drop in blood cell counts, including white cells – this means you can pick up infections more easily. Tell your doctor or nurse, or call your hospital advice line, if you have any side effects or feel generally unwell.

CAR T-cell therapy

CAR T- cell therapy is a new type of immunotherapy that is available on the NHS for some people with B cell ALL. Doctors may use it to treat people aged 25 or under with ALL that has come back or is no longer responding to treatment (relapsed or refractory ALL). T cells are a type of white blood cell that moves around the body to find and destroy defective cells. When you come into contact with a new infection or disease, the body makes T cells to fight that specific infection or disease. With CAR T-cell therapy, a specialist collects and makes a small change to your T cells. These cells are put back into your bloodstream and can target the cancer cells. This is a new and very specialist treatment and doctors are still learning about the side effects.

Types of targeted cancer drugs and immunotherapy for ALL

Imatinib (Glivec)

Imatinib is a targeted cancer drug (biological therapy) and is also known by its brand name Glivec (pronounced glee-vec).

It is a treatment for many different types of cancer.

How it works

Imatinib is a type of cancer growth blocker called a tyrosine kinase inhibitor (TKI). Tyrosine kinases are proteins that cells use to signal to each other to grow. They act as chemical messengers. There are a number of different tyrosine kinases and blocking them stops the cancer cells growing. Imatinib targets different tyrosine kinases, depending on the type of cancer.

How you have it

You have imatinib as a tablet that you swallow whole, with a glass of water after food. If you can't swallow the tablets, you can dissolve them in a glass of mineral water or apple juice. Drop the whole tablets into the fluid, and stir with a spoon until the tablets have broken up completely. Then drink the whole glassful.

Taking your tablets

- You must take tablets according to the instructions your doctor or pharmacist gives you.
- Speak to your pharmacist if you have problems swallowing the tablets.
- Whether you have a full or an empty stomach can affect how much of a drug gets into your bloodstream.

You should take the right dose, no more or less. Talk to your specialist or advice line before you stop taking a cancer drug.

When you have it

You have imatinib either once or twice a day, depending on the condition you have. You usually continue taking imatinib for as long as it works, unless the side effects get too bad. For acute lymphoblastic leukaemia that is Philadelphia chromosome positive, you may have imatinib on its own, or with chemotherapy.

Tests

You have blood tests before and during your treatment.

They check your levels of blood cells and other substances in the blood. They also check how well your liver and kidneys are working.

Side effects

We haven't listed all the side effects. It's very unlikely that you will have all of these side effects, but you might have some of them at the same time. How often and how severe the side effects are can vary from person to person. They also depend on what other treatments you're having. For example, your side effects could be worse if you're also having other drugs or radiotherapy.

When to contact your team

Your doctor, nurse or pharmacist will go through the possible side effects. They will monitor you closely during treatment and check how you are at your appointments. Contact your advice line as soon as possible if:

- ☐ you have severe side effects
- ☐ your side effects aren't getting any better
- ☐ your side effects are getting worse

Early treatment can help manage side effects better.

Contact your doctor or nurse immediately if you have signs of infection, including a temperature above 37.5C or below 36C.

Common side effects

Each of these effects happens in more than 10 in 100 people (10%). You might have one or more of them. They include:

Increased risk of getting an infection

Increased risk of getting an infection is due to a drop in white blood cells. Symptoms include a change in temperature, aching muscles, headaches, feeling cold and shivery and generally unwell. You might have other symptoms depending on where the infection is. Infections can sometimes be life threatening. You should contact your advice line urgently if you think you have an infection.

Breathlessness and looking pale

You might be breathless and look pale due to a drop in red blood cells. This is called anaemia.

Bruising, bleeding gums or nosebleeds

This is due to a drop in the number of platelets in your blood. These blood cells help the blood to clot when we cut ourselves. You may have nosebleeds or bleeding gums after brushing your teeth. Or you may have lots of tiny red spots or bruises on your arms or legs (known as petechia).

Tiredness and weakness (fatigue)

Tiredness and weakness (fatigue) can happen during and after treatment - doing gentle exercises each day can keep your energy up. Don't push yourself, rest when you start to feel tired and ask others for help.

Fluid build-up (oedema)

A build-up of fluid may cause swelling in your arms, hands, ankles, legs, face and other parts of the body. Contact your doctor if this happens to you.

Feeling or being sick

Feeling or being sick is usually well controlled with anti-sickness medicines. Avoiding fatty or fried foods, eating small meals and snacks, drinking plenty of water, and relaxation techniques, can all help.

Diarrhoea

Contact your advice line if you have diarrhoea, such as if you've had 4 or more loose watery poos (stools) in 24 hours. Or if you can't drink to replace the lost fluid. Or if it carries on for more than 3 days. Your doctor may give you anti diarrhoea medicine to take home with you after treatment. Eat less fibre, avoid raw fruits, fruit juice, cereals and vegetables, and drink plenty to replace the fluid lost.

Headaches

Tell your doctor or nurse if you keep getting headaches. They can give you painkillers to help.

Indigestion

Contact your doctor or pharmacist if you have indigestion or heartburn. They can prescribe medicines to help.

Skin rash

Skin problems include a skin rash, dry skin and itching. This usually goes back to normal when your treatment finishes. Your nurse will tell you what products you can use on your skin to help.

Muscle and joint pain

You might feel some pain from your muscles and joints. Speak to your doctor or nurse about what painkillers you can take to help with this.

Weight gain

You may gain weight while having this treatment. You may be able to control it with diet and exercise. Tell your doctor or nurse if you are finding it difficult to control your weight.

Tummy (abdominal) pain

Tell your treatment team if you have this. They can check the cause and give you medicine to help.

Occasional side effects

Each of these effects happens in more than 1 in 100 people (1%). You might have one or more of them. They include:

- constipation
- sore mouth
- liver changes
- taste changes
- weight loss

- dizziness
- difficulty sleeping (insomnia)
- sore eyes
- blurred vision
- loss of appetite
- wind (flatulence)
- numbness in hands or feet
- high temperature (fever)
- hair thinning
- cough

Rare side effects

These side effects happen in fewer than 1 in 100 people (1%). You might have one or more of them. They include:

- fluid around the heart (pericardial effusion)
- breast pain
- high uric acid levels in your body due to the breakdown of tumour cells (tumour lysis syndrome) - you have regular blood tests to check for this and may have a tablet called allopurinol to take

Other medicines, foods and drink

Cancer drugs can interact with some other medicines and herbal products. Tell your doctor or pharmacist about any medicines you are taking. This includes vitamins, herbal supplements and over the counter remedies.

Pregnancy and contraception

This treatment might harm a baby developing in the womb. It is important not to become pregnant or father a child while you're having treatment and for a few months afterwards. Talk to your doctor or nurse about effective contraception before starting treatment.

Fertility

You may not be able to become pregnant or father a child after treatment with this drug. Talk to your doctor before starting treatment if you think you may want to have a baby in the future. Men may be able to store sperm before starting treatment. Women may be able to store eggs or ovarian tissue but this is rare.

Breastfeeding

Don't breastfeed during this treatment because the drug may come through into your breast milk.

Treatment for other conditions

Always tell other doctors, nurses, pharmacists or dentists that you're having this treatment if you need treatment for anything else, including teeth problems.

Immunisations

Don't have immunisations with live vaccines while you're having treatment and for up to 12 months afterwards. The length of time depends on the treatment you are having. Ask your doctor or pharmacist how long you should avoid live vaccinations. In the UK, live vaccines include rubella, mumps, measles, BCG, yellow fever and the shingles vaccine (Zostavax).

You can:

- have other vaccines, but they might not give you as much protection as usual
- have the flu vaccine (as an injection)
- be in contact with other people who have had live vaccines as injections
- Avoid close contact with people who have recently had live vaccines taken by mouth (oral vaccines) such as oral polio or the typhoid vaccine.

This also includes the rotavirus vaccine given to babies. The virus is in the baby's poo for up to 2 weeks and could make you ill. So avoid changing their nappies for 2 weeks after their vaccination if possible. Or wear disposable gloves and wash your hands well afterwards. You should also avoid close contact with children who have had the flu vaccine nasal spray if your immune system is severely weakened.

Children and adolescents

Some children and adolescents taking imatinib may have slower than normal growth. The treatment team will monitor this carefully.

Dasatinib (Sprycel)

- Dasatinib is pronounced das-at-in-nib and is also known by its brand name Sprycel.
- Dasatinib is a treatment for:
- chronic myeloid leukaemia
- acute myeloid leukaemia which is Philadelphia chromosome positive, when other treatments are no longer working
- acute lymphoblastic leukaemia which is Philadelphia chromosome positive, when other treatments are no longer working

It is also being used in clinical trials for other types of cancer.

How it works

Dasatinib is a type of drug called a protein tyrosine kinase inhibitor (TKI). Tyrosine kinases are proteins that act as chemical messengers to stimulate cancer cells to grow. Dasatinib blocks the tyrosine kinases from sending chemical signals that tell the cells to grow.

How you have it

You have dasatinib as tablets. You swallow them whole with a glass of water. You can take them with or without food. You have dasatinib either once or twice a day. You usually carry on taking it for as long as it works, unless the side effects get too bad.

If you are taking any medicines for indigestion (antacids), take them either 2 hours before or 2 hours after the dasatinib. These medicines can stop the body absorbing dasatinib. You should not take any other medicines that affect the production of stomach acid.

Taking your tablets

- ☐ Your doctor will tell you how many tablets to take.
- ☐ You should take the right dose, not more or less.
- ☐ Never stop taking a cancer drug without talking to your specialist first.
- ☐ You need to take your tablets according to the instructions your doctor or pharmacist gives you.

Tests

You have blood tests before and during your treatment. They check your levels of blood cells and other substances in the blood. They also check how well your liver and kidneys are working.

Side effects

We haven't listed all the side effects. It's very unlikely that you will have all of these side effects, but you might have some of them at the same time. How often and how severe the side effects are can vary from person to person. They also depend on what other treatments you're having. For example, your side effects could be worse if you're also having other drugs or radiotherapy.

When to contact your team

Your doctor, nurse or pharmacist will go through the possible side effects. They will monitor you closely during treatment and check how you are at your appointments. Contact your advice line as soon as possible if:

- you have severe side effects
- your side effects aren't getting any better
- your side effects are getting worse
- Early treatment can help manage side effects better.

Contact your doctor or nurse immediately if you have signs of infection, including a temperature above 37.5C or below 36C.

Common side effects

These side effects happen in more than 10 in 100 people (10%). You might have one or more of them. They include:

Increased risk of getting an infection

Increased risk of getting an infection is due to a drop in white blood cells. Symptoms include a change in temperature, aching muscles, headaches, feeling cold and shivery and generally unwell. You might have other symptoms depending on where the infection is.Infections can sometimes be life threatening. You should contact your advice line urgently if you think you have an infection.

Berathlessness and looking pale

You might be breathless and look pale due to a drop in red

blood cells. This is called anaemia.

Bruising, bleeding gums or nosebleeds

This is due to a drop in the number of platelets in your blood. These blood cells help the blood to clot when we cut ourselves. You may have nosebleeds or bleeding gums after brushing your teeth. Or you may have lots of tiny red spots or bruises on your arms or legs (known as petechia).

Diarrhoea

Contact your advice line if you have diarrhoea, such as if you've had 4 or more loose watery poos (stools) in 24 hours. Or if you can't drink to replace the lost fluid. Or if it carries on for more than 3 days. Your doctor may give you anti diarrhoea medicine to take home with you after treatment. Eat less fibre, avoid raw fruits, fruit juice, cereals and vegetables, and drink plenty to replace the fluid lost.

Headaches

Tell your doctor or nurse if you keep getting headaches. They can give you painkillers to help.

- Fluid around the lungs (pleural effusion)
- Talk to the team looking after you if you are breathless.

Skin changes

Skin problems include a skin rash, dry skin and itching. This usually goes back to normal when your treatment finishes. Your nurse will tell you what products you can use on your skin to help.

Fluid build-up (oedema)

A build-up of fluid may cause swelling in your arms, hands, ankles, legs, face and other parts of the body. Contact your doctor if this happens to you.

☐ Tiredness and weakness (fatigue)

☐ You might feel very tired and as though you lack energy.

Various things can help you to reduce tiredness and cope with it, for example exercise. Some research has shown that taking gentle exercise can give you more energy. It is important to balance exercise with resting.

Feeling or being sick

Feeling or being sick is usually well controlled with anti-sickness medicines. Avoiding fatty or fried foods, eating small meals and snacks, drinking plenty of water, and relaxation techniques, can all help.

Bone or muscle pain

You might feel some pain from your muscles and joints. Speak to your doctor or nurse about what painkillers you can take to help with this.

Occasional side effects

These side effects happen in between 1 and 10 out of every 100 people (1 to 10%). You might have one or more of them. They include:

☐ numbness or tingling in fingers or toes

☐ indigestion

- loss of appetite
- sore mouth
- hair loss
- dizziness
- ringing in the ears (tinnitus)
- eye problems
- aching and stiff muscles and joints
- difficulty sleeping (insomnia)
- depression
- general weakness
- weight changes
- chills
- increased blood pressure
- flushing
- chest pain

Rare side effects

These side effects happen in fewer than 1 in 100 people (1%). You might have one or more of them. They include:

- confusion or memory changes
- heart problems
- low levels of thyroid hormones
- dehydration
- changes in mineral levels in the blood
- anxiety

- loss of interest in sex
- bleeding in the brain
- hearing loss
- balance changes (vertigo)
- liver changes
- growth of breast tissue in men (gynecomastia)
- periods stopping

Coping with side effects

We have more information about side effects and tips on how to cope with them.

Other medicines, foods and drink

Cancer drugs can interact with some other medicines and herbal products. Tell your doctor or pharmacist about any medicines you are taking. This includes vitamins, herbal supplements and over the counter remedies.

Pregnancy and contraception

This treatment might harm a baby developing in the womb. It is important not to become pregnant or father a child while you're having treatment and for a few months afterwards. Talk to your doctor or nurse about effective contraception before starting treatment.

Fertility

It is not known whether this treatment affects fertility in people. Talk to your doctor before starting treatment if you think you may want to have a baby in the future.

Breastfeeding

Don't breastfeed during this treatment because the drug may come through into your breast milk.

Treatment for other conditions

Always tell other doctors, nurses, pharmacists or dentists that you're having this treatment if you need treatment for anything else, including teeth problems.

Immunisations

Don't have immunisations with live vaccines while you're having treatment and for up to 12 months afterwards. The length of time depends on the treatment you are having. Ask your doctor or pharmacist how long you should avoid live vaccinations. In the UK, live vaccines include rubella, mumps, measles, BCG, yellow fever and the shingles vaccine (Zostavax).

You can:

- have other vaccines, but they might not give you as much protection as usual
- have the flu vaccine (as an injection)
- be in contact with other people who have had live vaccines as injections
- Avoid close contact with people who have recently had live vaccines taken by mouth (oral vaccines) such as oral polio or the typhoid vaccine.

This also includes the rotavirus vaccine given to babies. The virus is in the baby's poo for up to 2 weeks and could make you ill. So avoid changing their nappies for 2 weeks after their vaccination if possible. Or wear disposable gloves and wash your hands well afterwards.

You should also avoid close contact with children who have had the flu vaccine nasal spray if your immune system is severely weakened.

Ponatinib (Iclusig)

- Ponatinib is a type of targeted cancer drug. It is also called by its brand name Iclusig. You might have it as a treatment for:
- chronic myeloid leukaemia where the leukaemic cells have gene change (mutation) called T315I
- acute lymphoblastic leukaemia that has an abnormal chromosome called the Philadelphia chromosome, or has the T315I mutation

You may also have it as part of clinical trials for other cancers.

How it works

Ponatinib is a type of drug called a protein tyrosine kinase inhibitor (TKI). Tyrosine kinases are proteins that act as chemical messengers to stimulate cancer cells to grow. Ponatinib blocks and interferes with a number of protein kinases. It is called a multi kinase inhibitor.

How you have it

Ponatinib comes as tablets. You swallow the tablets whole with a glass of water once a day. You can take them with or without food.

Taking your tablets or capsules

You must take tablets and capsules according to the instructions your doctor or pharmacist gives you.

You should take the right dose, not more or less. Never stop taking a cancer drug without talking to your specialist first.

When you have it

You usually carry on taking ponatinib for as long as it works, unless the side effects get too bad.

Tests

You have blood tests before and during your treatment. They check your levels of blood cells and other substances in the blood. They also check how well your liver and kidneys are working.

Side effects

We haven't listed all the side effects. It's very unlikely that you will have all of these side effects, but you might have some of them at the same time. How often and how severe the side effects are can vary from person to person. They also depend on what other treatments you're having. For example, your side effects could be worse if you're also having other drugs or radiotherapy.

When to contact your team

Your doctor, nurse or pharmacist will go through the possible side effects. They will monitor you closely during treatment and check how you are at your appointments. Contact your advice line as soon as possible if:

- you have severe side effects
- your side effects aren't getting any better
- your side effects are getting worse
- Early treatment can help manage side effects better.

Contact your doctor or nurse immediately if you have signs of infection, including a temperature above 37.5C or below 36C.

Common side effects

Each of these effects happens in more than 1 in 10 people (10%). You might have one or more of them. They include:

Increased risk of getting an infection

Increased risk of getting an infection is due to a drop in white blood cells. Symptoms include a change in temperature, aching muscles, headaches, feeling cold and shivery and generally unwell. You might have other symptoms depending on where the infection is. Infections can sometimes be life threatening. You should contact your advice line urgently if you think you have an infection.

Breathless and looking pale

You might be breathless and look pale due to a drop in red blood cells. This is called anaemia.

Bruising, bleeding gums or nosebleeds

This is due to a drop in the number of platelets in your blood. These blood cells help the blood to clot when we cut ourselves. You may have nosebleeds or bleeding gums after brushing your teeth. Or you may have lots of tiny red spots or bruises on your arms or legs (known as petechia).

Skin changes

Skin problems include a skin rash, dry skin and itching. This usually goes back to normal when your treatment finishes. Your nurse will tell you what products you can use on your skin to help.

Pain

You might feel some pain from your muscles and joints. Speak to your doctor or nurse about what painkillers you can take to help with this.

Headaches

Tell your doctor or nurse if you keep getting headaches. They can give you painkillers to help.

Dizziness

This drug may make you feel drowsy or dizzy. Don't drive or operate machinery if you have this.

High blood pressure

Tell your doctor or nurse if you have headaches, nose bleeds, blurred or double vision or shortness of breath. Your nurse will check your blood pressure regularly.

Cough

You might develop a cough or breathing problems. This could be due to infection, such as pneumonia or inflammation of the lungs (pneumonitis). Let your doctor or nurse know straight away if you suddenly become breathless or develop a cough.

Loss of appetite

You might lose your appetite for various reasons when you are having cancer treatment. Sickness, taste changes or tiredness can put you off food and drinks.

Difficulty sleeping

It can help to change a few things about how you try to sleep. Try to go to bed and get up at the same time each day and spend some time relaxing before you go to bed. Some light exercise each day may also help.

Tiredness and weakness (fatigue)

You might feel very tired and as though you lack energy. Various things can help you to reduce tiredness and cope with it, for example exercise. Some research has shown that taking gentle exercise can give you more energy. It is important to balance exercise with resting.

Feeling or being sick

Feeling or being sick is usually well controlled with anti-sickness medicines. Avoiding fatty or fried foods, eating small meals and snacks, drinking plenty of water, and relaxation techniques, can all help.

Fluid build-up (swelling)

This usually goes away on its own, but tell your doctor or nurse if you have it.

Constipation

Constipation is easier to sort out if you treat it early. Drink plenty of fluids and eat as much fresh fruit and vegetables as you can. Try to take gentle exercise, such as walking. Tell your doctor or nurse if you are constipated for more than 3 days. They can prescribe a laxative.

Diarrhoea

Contact your advice line if you have diarrhoea, such as if you've had 4 or more loose watery poos (stools) in 24 hours. Or if you can't drink to replace the lost fluid. Or if it carries on for more than 3 days. Your doctor may give you anti diarrhoea medicine to take home with you after treatment. Eat less fibre, avoid raw fruits, fruit juice, cereals and vegetables, and drink plenty to replace the fluid lost.

Occasional side effects

Each of these effects happens in more than 1 in 100 people (1%). You might have one or more of them. They include:

- Flu symptoms
- inflammation of the pancreas (pancreatitis)
- heart problems
- weight loss
- dehydration
- increased risk of stroke
- numbness or tingling in the hands or feet
- blood clots
- fluid on the lungs
- voice changes
- eye problems
- problems getting an erection
- liver changes
- change in blood sugar (glucose) levels
- low levels of thyroid hormones

Rare side effects

Each of these effects happens in fewer than 1 in 100 people (1%). You might have one or more of them. They include:

- yellow skin and eyes (jaundice)
- a stomach bleed
- high uric acid levels in the blood due to the breaking down of cancer cells

Possible long term side effects

Ponatinib is a fairly new drug in cancer treatment. This means that there is limited information available at the moment about possible longer term effects that it may cause. Tell your doctor if you notice anything that is not normal for you.

Other medicines, foods and drinks

Cancer drugs can interact with some other medicines and herbal products. Tell your doctor or pharmacist about any medicines you are taking. This includes vitamins, herbal supplements and over the counter remedies. Some medicines, foods and herbal supplements that contain CYP enzymes can interfere with how ponatinib works. Speak to your doctor about this. You should not eat grapefruit or drink grapefruit juice when you are taking this drug because it can react with the drug.

Pregnancy and contraception

This treatment might harm a baby developing in the womb. It is important not to become pregnant or father a child while you're having treatment and for a few months afterwards. Talk to your doctor or nurse about effective contraception before starting treatment.

Breastfeeding

Don't breastfeed during this treatment because the drug may come through into your breast milk.

Fertility

You may not be able to become pregnant or father a child after treatment with this drug. Talk to your doctor before starting treatment if you think you may want to have a baby in the future. Men may be able to store sperm before starting treatment. Women may be able to store eggs or ovarian tissue but this is rare.

Treatment for other conditions

Always tell other doctors, nurses, pharmacists or dentists that you're having this treatment if you need treatment for anything else, including teeth problems.

Immunisations

Don't have immunisations with live vaccines while you're having treatment and for up to 12 months afterwards. The length of time depends on the treatment you are having. Ask your doctor or pharmacist how long you should avoid live vaccinations. In the UK, live vaccines include rubella, mumps, measles, BCG, yellow fever and the shingles vaccine (Zostavax).

You can:

- have other vaccines, but they might not give you as much protection as usual
- have the flu vaccine (as an injection)
- be in contact with other people who have had live vaccines as injections

Avoid close contact with people who have recently had live vaccines taken by mouth (oral vaccines) such as oral polio or the typhoid vaccine. This also includes the rotavirus vaccine given to babies. The virus is in the baby's poo for up to 2 weeks and could make you ill. So avoid changing their nappies for 2 weeks after their vaccination if possible. Or wear disposable gloves and wash your hands well afterwards. You should also avoid close contact with children who have had the flu vaccine nasal spray if your immune system is severely weakened.

Radiotherapy

Radiotherapy means the use of radiation, usually x-rays, to treat cancer. You might have radiotherapy as part of your treatment for acute lymphoblastic leukaemia (ALL). You might have radiotherapy to the brain or spinal cord if leukaemia cells have spread there. Or you might have radiotherapy to the whole body as part of a stem cell transplant.

Planning radiotherapy

Radiotherapy means the use of radiation, usually x-rays, to destroy cancer cells. You might have external radiotherapy as part of your treatment for ALL. External radiotherapy uses a machine outside the body to aim radiation beams at the cancer. Before you start treatment, your radiotherapy team has to carefully plan it. This means working out how much radiation you need and exactly where you need it. You have a planning appointment, which takes from 15 minutes to 2 hours. You have a CT scan in the radiotherapy department to help with planning.

Your radiographers tell you what is going to happen. They help you into position on the scan couch. You might have a type of firm cushion called a vacbag to help you keep still.

The CT scanner couch is the same type of bed that you lie on for your treatment sessions. You need to lie very still. Tell your radiographers if you aren't comfortable.

Injection of dye

You might need an injection of contrast into a vein in your hand. This is a dye that helps body tissues show up more clearly on the scan.

Before you have the contrast, your radiographer asks you about any medical conditions or allergies. Some people are allergic to the contrast.

Having the scan

Once you are in position your radiographers put some markers on your skin. They move the couch up and through the scanner. They then leave the room and the scan starts. The scan takes about 5 minutes. You won't feel anything. Your radiographers can see and hear you from the CT control area where they operate the scanner. If you are going to have radiotherapy to the brain or top or your spinal cord, your radiographer or a technician might make a mask for you before you have the planning CT scan. The mask is to help keep you still and in the correct position during your treatment.

Radiotherapy treatment mask

Your radiographer or technician makes your mask in the

radiotherapy department. They might call the mask a radiotherapy shell. The mask covers your face, and the top and sides of your head. It attaches to the couch when you are lying down for the planning scan or radiotherapy treatment. The process of making the mask can vary slightly between hospitals. It usually takes around 30 minutes.

Before making the mask

You need to wear clothes that you can easily take off from your neck and chest. You also need to take off any jewellery from that area. Facial hair, long hair or dreadlocks can make it difficult to mould the mask. Your radiotherapy team will tell you if you need to shave or tie your hair back.

Making the mask

The technician uses a special kind of plastic that they heat in warm water. This makes it soft and pliable. They put the plastic on to your face so that it moulds exactly. It feels a little like a warm flannel and is a mesh with holes in so you can breathe. After a few minutes the mesh gets hard. The technician takes the mask off and it cools down. You might need to have one more fitting to make sure it is exactly right. You wear the mask for your planning CT scan. Your radiotherapy team keep the mask in the department for when you go back for treatment. You wear it for each treatment session

C:\Users\CC LEEDS\Downloads\rrrrrrrr.png

Your radiographers tell you what is going to happen. They help you into position on the scan couch. You might have a type of firm cushion called a vacbag to help you keep still.

The CT scanner couch is the same type of bed that you lie on for your treatment sessions. You need to lie very still. Tell your radiographers if you aren't comfortable.

Injection of dye

You might need an injection of contrast into a vein in your hand. This is a dye that helps body tissues show up more clearly on the scan. Before you have the contrast, your radiographer asks you about any medical conditions or allergies. Some people are allergic to the contrast.

Having the scan

Once you are in position your radiographers put some markers on your skin. They move the couch up and through the scanner. They then leave the room and the scan starts. The scan takes about 5 minutes. You won't feel anything. Your radiographers can see and hear you from the CT control area where they operate the scanner. If you are going to have radiotherapy to the brain or top or your spinal cord, your radiographer or a technician might make a mask for you before you have the planning CT scan. The mask is to help keep you still and in the correct position during your treatment.

Radiotherapy treatment mask (shell)

Your radiographer or technician makes your mask in the radiotherapy department. They might call the mask a radiotherapy shell. The mask covers your face, and the top and sides of your head. It attaches to the couch when you are lying down for the planning scan or radiotherapy treatment. The process of making the mask can vary slightly between hospitals. It usually takes around 30 minutes.

Before making the mask

You need to wear clothes that you can easily take off from your neck and chest. You also need to take off any jewellery from that area. Facial hair, long hair or dreadlocks can make it difficult to mould the mask. Your radiotherapy team will tell you if you need to shave or tie your hair back.

Making the mask

The technician uses a special kind of plastic that they heat in warm water. This makes it soft and pliable. They put the plastic on to your face so that it moulds exactly. It feels a little like a warm flannel and is a mesh with holes in so you can breathe. After a few minutes the mesh gets hard. The technician takes the mask off and it cools down. You might need to have one more fitting to make sure it is exactly right. You wear the mask for your planning CT scan. Your radiotherapy team keep the mask in the department for when you go back for treatment. You wear it for each treatment session.

C:\Users\CC LEEDS\Downloads\ffffffffff.png

Radiotherapy planning for TBI

You might have radiotherapy as part of a stem cell transplant. In this case you have radiotherapy to your whole body. This is called total body irradiation (TBI).First you have a planning session of about an hour to create the treatment plan. You usually lie on your back on the couch. You might have your arms across your chest or resting on your lower tummy (abdomen). Your radiographers will put support pads (cushions) under your knees and you might also have supportive pads around your body to keep you in position. Your radiographers take several measurements and then you have a CT scan. They will make two very small permanent dots on both sides of your hips. They use these marks to help put you in the correct position when you have your treatment. During this session you might have a very small dose of radiotherapy. This is to help with the planning. You have no side effects from this.

Total body irradiation

After your planning session

Your radiographer will tell you when to go back for your treatment sessions. It takes at least a few days for your radiotherapy team to create your radiotherapy plan.

Radiotherapy to the brain

Radiotherapy uses radiation, usually x-rays, to treat cancer. You might have radiotherapy to treat leukaemia cells that have spread to the brain or spinal cord.

Before treatment

Before your radiotherapy, you have a planning session which includes having a CT scan. You often also have a mask made that keeps your head very still and in the correct position while you have treatment.

The radiotherapy room

Radiotherapy machines are very big. They rotate around you to give you your treatment. The machine doesn't touch you at any point. Before you start your course of treatment your radiographers explain what you will see and hear. In some departments the treatment rooms have docks for you to plug in your music player. So you can listen to your own music.

C:\Users\CC LEEDS\Downloads\vvvvvvvvvvvv.png

Before each treatment

Your radiographers help you to get into position on the radiotherapy table. If you need to wear a mask for your radiotherapy, they will position the mask over your face and attach it to the table. The mask keeps your head completely still while you have treatment. The room is darkened and your radiographers line you up in the radiotherapy machine using laser lights and the marks on the mask or your skin. You will hear them saying measurements to each other to get you in the right position. They then leave you alone in the room for a few minutes.

During the treatment

You need to lie very still on your back. Your radiographers might take images (x-rays or scans) before your treatment to make sure that you're in the right position. The machine makes whirring and beeping sounds. You won't feel anything when you have the treatment. Your radiographers can see and hear you on a CCTV screen in the next room. They can talk to you over an intercom and might ask you to hold your breath or take shallow breaths at times. You can also talk to them through the intercom or raise your hand if you need to stop or if you're uncomfortable.

Side effects

You will have some side effects during treatment and for a few weeks afterwards. These include:

- ☐ Feeling or being sick
- ☐ Tiredness
- ☐ Hair loss
- ☐ Skin changes
- ☐ Headaches
- ☐ Hearing problems

Possible long term side effects

Some people have long term side effects. These can include:

- ☐ Cataracts
- ☐ Skin sensitivity to the sun
- ☐ Small risk of a second cancer

Total body radiotherapy (TBI)

Radiotherapy uses radiation, usually x-rays, to treat cancer cells. You might have radiotherapy to your whole body before a stem cell transplant. This is called total body irradiation or TBI. You also have chemotherapy. The aim of this intensive treatment is to kill the leukaemia cells. It also destroys your immune system. This means that after your transplant your body is less likely to reject the new healthy stem cells and they can grow. You usually have TBI twice a day for 3 or 4 days, or as a single treatment.

The radiotherapy room

Radiotherapy machines are very big. They rotate around you to give you your treatment. The machine doesn't touch you at any point. Before you start your course of treatment your radiographers explain what you will see and hear. In some departments the treatment rooms have docks for you to plug in your music player. So you can listen to your own music.

Before treatment

You have a planning session a week or two before your first treatment. It takes around an hour. This session is for your radiotherapy team to carefully plan your radiotherapy and work out what shielding you need to make sure your whole body receives the same amount of radiation.

During treatment

Your nurse gives you anti sickness medicines about half an hour before the treatment. In the radiotherapy room, the radiographers help you to get into position on the radiotherapy table. They darken the room and line you up in the radiotherapy machine using laser lights and marks on your skin. You will hear them saying measurements to each other to get you in the right position. They attach devices over your clothes that measure the treatment dose to various parts of your body. Then your radiographers leave you alone in the room for 10 to 15 minutes while you have the treatment. They can still see and hear you. You must lie very still and not move. Afterwards, your radiographers come back into the room to turn the radiotherapy couch. You then have treatment for another 10 to 15 minutes to treat the other side of your body.

After treatment

You go back to the ward after each treatment. In between treatments you must stay away from anyone who may be unwell. Your white blood cell count will be very low, so it is easy for your body to pick up an infection. Once you have finished the course of radiotherapy, you have the stem cell transplant through a drip into your bloodstream. This happens as an inpatient on the ward.

Side effects

Total body irradiation causes side effects. These may happen shortly after treatment, or months or years afterwards (long term effects). Your radiotherapy team will talk to you about the possible side effects before you start treatment. Let your doctor or nurse know straight away if you get any side effects.

Early side effects include:

- Skin changes
- Hair loss
- Feeling sick or being sick
- Tiredness
- Diarrhoea
- A dry mouth
- Risk of infection
- Sore mouth

Possible long term effects

Some side effects can happen weeks, months or years after the treatment. Long term side effects include:

- ☐ Cataracts
- ☐ Lung inflammation
- ☐ Infertility

Growth factors

Growth factors are natural substances that stimulate the bone marrow to make blood cells. Some growth factors are used during chemotherapy treatment.

When you have growth factors

You might have growth factors in the following situations:

After chemotherapy

Your white blood cell count drops after having chemotherapy and so you are at an increased risk of getting an infection. The longer your white cell count is low the greater your risk. Having a growth factor helps your white cell count go up more quickly. This could lower the risk of infection.

Before stem cell collection for a transplant

Growth factors are given before collecting stem cells for a stem cell transplant. Stem cells develop into blood cells, such as white blood cells. Daily growth factor injections make the bone marrow produce many more stem cells than normal. These extra stem cells spill over into the bloodstream. They are then collected by a machine. You have the stem cells through a drip after having high dose chemotherapy. In ALL, most stem cells are collected from a donor.

How you have growth factors

You usually have growth factors as an injection under the skin. This might be in the tummy (abdomen), or into an arm or a leg. You have the injections every day. How long you have them for depends on why you are having them. Your nurse or doctor will talk to you about this. You might have growth factors through a drip into your bloodstream (intravenously) after having a transplant.

Growth factor type

Doctors sometimes use the growth factor called granulocyte colony stimulating factor or G-CSF during ALL treatment.

There are different types of G-CSF called:

- ☐ filgrastim
- ☐ lenograstim

- pegfilgrastim- this is a long acting type

Side effects

Common side effects of growth factors include:
- itching around the injection site
- pain in your bones
- fever

Stem cell or bone marrow transplants

You have a transplant after high dose chemotherapy and sometimes radiotherapy. The transplant is sometimes called a stem cell or bone marrow rescue.

What is a stem cell or bone marrow transplant?

You might have a stem cell or bone marrow transplant as part of your treatment for acute lymphoblastic leukaemia (ALL). A transplant allows you to have high doses of chemotherapy and other treatments. The stem cells are collected from the bloodstream or the bone marrow.

What are stem cells?

Stem cells are very early cells made in the bone marrow. Bone marrow is a spongy material that fills the bones.

These stem cells develop into red blood cells, white blood cells and platelets.

Red blood cells contain haemoglobin which carries oxygen around the body. White blood cells are part of your immune system and help to fight infection. Platelets help to clot the blood to prevent bleeding.

How transplants work

To prepare you for a stem cell transplant you usually have very high doses of chemotherapy first. You might have other treatment as well. This might be radiotherapy to the whole body (total body irradiation or TBI), or targeted cancer drugs, or both. This preparation is also known as conditioning treatment. The treatment kills the leukaemia cells as well as the healthy stem cells in your bone marrow. This makes space in your bone marrow for the donor stem cells. And dampens down your immune system so you don't reject the donor cells.

Before your high dose chemotherapy, your team either collects:

☐ someone else's (donor) stem cells

☐ your own stem cells (this is very rare in ALL)

After the conditioning treatment you have the stem cells

into your bloodstream through a drip. The cells find their way back to your bone marrow. You start making blood cells again and your bone marrow slowly recovers.

A stem cell or bone marrow transplant

The main difference between a stem cell and bone marrow transplant is whether stem cells are collected from the bloodstream or bone marrow. A stem cell transplant uses stem cells from a donor's bloodstream or your bloodstream. This is also called a peripheral blood stem cell transplant (PBSCT). A bone marrow transplant uses stem cells from a donor's bone marrow or your bone marrow. Stem cell transplants are the most common type of transplant. Bone marrow transplants are not used as much. This is because:

- it's easier to collect stem cells from the bloodstream than bone marrow
- the treatment team can usually collect more cells from the bloodstream
- blood cell levels tend to recover quicker after a stem cell transplant

Giving stem cells rather than bone marrow is better for the donor. They don't need an anaesthetic for the stem cell collection and tend to recover more quickly. Your doctor will explain how they have decided what kind of transplant is best for you.

Why you might have a transplant

The aim of treatment is to put it into complete remission. Complete remission means there is no sign of leukaemia cells.

Your doctor might suggest a transplant if your ALL:

☐ has features that show it is likely to come back (high risk)

☐ has comes back (relapsed ALL)

Types of transplant

You usually have stem cells from another person (a donor) in acute lymphoblastic leukaemia (ALL). This is called an allogeneic transplant or allograft.

You might have stem cells from:

☐ a brother or sister (sibling match)

☐ a person unrelated to you whose stem cells are similar to yours (matched unrelated donor or MUD)

☐ cord blood stem cells (umbilical cord)

Usually, the team collects stem cells from your donor's bloodstream (peripheral blood stem cell harvest). But occasionally they collect the stem cells directly from the donor's bone marrow. You might have a stem cell transplant using stem cells from umbilical cord blood. Doctors take blood from the umbilical cord and placenta that is very rich in stem cells. The blood bank may give the donated stem cells to a person whose blood cells closely match the donated cells. Cord transplants are mostly used for children because a smaller amount of cells are collected. You could have a stem cell transplant from 2 different umbilical cords. This is called a double cord transplant.

Finding a donor

Your doctor can test your brothers or sisters if you have them to see if they are a match. Or they can search national and international databases to try to find an unrelated match. They see how many particular proteins on the surface of the cells match yours. This is called tissue typing or HLA matching. HLA stands for human leucocyte antigen.

> Find out more about donating stem cells
>
> Having your own stem cells (autologous stem cell transplant)
>
> You might have your own stem cells back after high dose treatment instead of using a donor's. But this is rare for ALL. This is called an autologous stem cell transplant or autograft.

Stages of a donor stem cell transplant

C:\Users\CC LEEDS\Downloads\ssssssss.png

Stages of a donor stem cell transplant

Preparation and finding a donor

Your medical team look for and test possible donors.

To prepare you for your transplant, you have various tests. Closer to the time of the transplant you have a central line put in if you haven't got one already. You might also need a feeding tube. You may have chemotherapy before your high dose treatment.

Donor's stem cell collection or harvest

Once your donor is found, the transplant team prepare them for their donation of stem cells. Your donor has injections of a growth factor if they are going to have stem cells collected from their bloodstream (peripheral blood stem cell collection). The growth factor makes the stem cells in the bone marrow spill out into the bloodstream. When there are enough stem cells, the transplant team collects them from their bloodstream. Your donor will need a general anaesthetic if they are having stem cells taken directly from their bone marrow. A doctor puts a needle into their hip bone to remove the bone marrow. Your high dose treatment and having your donor's cells

When a donor is found, you have high dose treatment also called conditioning treatment. This involves having high dose chemotherapy. You might also have whole body radiotherapy or a targeted cancer drug, or both. You then have the donor's stem cells through a drip into your bloodstream.

Blood count recovery

The stem cells find their way to your bone marrow where they start to make blood cells. This recovery of blood cells is called engraftment. Blood count recovery depends on the type of transplant you have. It can take around 2 weeks to see some blood count recovery with peripheral blood stem cells, 3 weeks with bone marrow stem cells and about 4 weeks with cord blood stem cells.

Collecting stem cells

You might have a stem cell or bone marrow transplant as part of your treatment for acute lymphoblastic leukaemia (ALL). Part of this process is collecting stem cells from the bloodstream or the bone marrow. Stem cells are made in the bone marrow and develop into red blood cells, white blood cells and platelets. In ALL, stem cells are usually collected from someone else (a donor). This is called an allogeneic transplant.

Collecting your donor's stem cells from the blood

This is called a peripheral blood stem cell collection or harvest. It is the most common way of collecting stem cells for a transplant.

Preparing for the stem cell collection

First, your donor has injections of a growth factor called G-CSF. They have the injections once a day for about 4 days. Growth factors are natural proteins that help the bone marrow to make blood cells. They make the bone marrow produce more stem cells so they spill out into the bloodstream. Your donor has a blood test the day after the last injection to make sure they have enough stem cells in their blood. They can then have the stem cell collection.

On collection day

Your donor might have their stem cells collected over 1 or 2 days. It takes about 4 hours each time. They lay down on a couch. The nurse puts a drip into each of their arms and attaches the drip to a machine. The blood passes out of one drip, through the machine, and back into their body through the other drip. The machine filters the stem cells out of their blood and collects them in a bag. You usually have the stem cells later the same day or the next day.

Side effects of a stem cell collection

During the stem cell collection your donor might have:

- tingling around their mouth
- muscle cramps

This happens if their calcium level gets low. They have extra calcium through a drip if this happens. They might feel very tired for a couple of days after having the stem cell collection.

- ☐ Collecting stem cells from your donor's bone marrow
- ☐ Collecting bone marrow is called a bone marrow harvest.

What happens

Your donor has a general anaesthetic. This means they are in a deep sleep during the procedure. The doctor puts a needle through their skin into the back of the hip bone. They pull the liquid bone marrow out through the needle into a syringe. They then inject it into a bag.

To get enough marrow the doctor usually puts the needle into several different parts of the hip bone. Occasionally, doctors use the breast bone (sternum) as well. The doctor removes about a litre (nearly 2 pints) of bone marrow. Your donor's body replaces these cells within a few weeks.

Recovery

When they wake up, they may have up to 6 puncture sites covered with dressings. They will feel very bruised and sore. This can last for up to a week, but painkillers can help. They usually stay in hospital overnight after a bone marrow harvest. This is to make sure they have recovered from the anaesthetic. They might need a blood transfusion afterwards.

Side effects of a transplant

The side effects of a transplant are usually worst just after chemotherapy and radiotherapy and for a few weeks afterwards.

The possible side effects of a transplant depend on your:

- treatment schedule
- type of transplant

High dose chemotherapy can have the same side effects as standard chemotherapy. You have the same chemotherapy drugs. But as you are having higher doses, the side effects might be more severe. You might have additional side effects if you also have radiotherapy to your whole body (total body irradiation).

Side effects of high dose chemotherapy

Chemotherapy side effects can start straight after your treatment and last for some time afterwards. When your blood counts start to rise you usually start to feel better.

Some side effects are serious and they can be life threatening. Let your team know if you have any side effects. They can do a lot to help you. Other side effects might affect you in the longer term. Let your team know about any side effects. They can help to relieve some of these:

- An increased risk of infection
- Anaemia
- Increased risk of bleeding or bruising
- Sickness and diarrhoea
- A sore mouth
- Difficulty eating and drinking
- Feeling tired and run down
- Hair loss

Side effects of radiotherapy

Treatment for ALL can include whole body radiotherapy. This is called total body irradiation (TBI). You have it after high dose chemotherapy, just before you have your stem cell or bone marrow transplant.

Radiotherapy side effects include:

- feeling or being sick
- tiredness and weakness (fatigue)
- diarrhoea
- problems with your thyroid (hypothyroidism)
- heart problems
- risk of second cancer
- hair loss

You might sleep a lot for a few days after the treatment. Your nurses make sure you have as much anti sickness medicine as you need. Do tell your nurses about sickness and diarrhoea so they can give you something to help control it.

Fertility

Infertility is a long term side effect of this type of treatment. Unfortunately most people can no longer have children after high dose treatment. This can be very difficult for some people to cope with. Sometimes men and teenage boys can store sperm before they start their chemotherapy, so that they can still father a child in the future. This is called sperm banking. Ask your doctor if you think you would like to do this. For women, chemotherapy can cause an early menopause. You might be able to have hormone replacement therapy (HRT) to treat the symptoms of a menopause. Ask your doctor about this. Sometimes women can freeze their eggs or embryos before they start treatment. Talk to your doctor early on if you want to find out more about this. It can take a few weeks to do this and may delay your cancer treatment. So it might not be possible. Your nurse will help support you with this.

Graft versus host disease

Graft versus host disease (GvHD) is a side effect of transplants from a relative or matched unrelated donor. GvHD happens because the donor stem cells contain cells from your donor's immune system. These cells sometimes recognise your own tissues as being foreign and attack them. This causes side effects, but can also be an advantage. This is because the immune cells might also attack any leukaemia cells left after your treatment.

GvHD can be acute or chronic.

Acute GvHD starts within 100 days of the transplant. It can cause:

- diarrhoea
- weight loss
- changes in the way your liver works
- skin rashes

Your doctor will give you drugs called immunosuppressants if you develop GvHD after your transplant. These drugs calm down this immune reaction.

Chronic GvHD starts more than 100 days after the transplant. With chronic GvHD you might have skin rashes, diarrhoea, sore joints and dry eyes. Your doctor will treat your symptoms with steroids and other drugs. They usually suggest that you stay out of the sun because it can make your skin rashes worse.

Side effects of treatment

Treatment for acute lymphoblastic leukaemia (ALL) might cause short and longer term side effects.

What side effects are

Side effects are unwanted things that happen to you as a result of medical treatment. The side effects that you might have and how severe they are depend on a number of factors including:

- the type of treatment you have
- the combination of treatments you have
- the dose (amount) of the drug or radiotherapy
- the way you have treatment – as tablets or capsules, or by injection
- your general health
- your age

Many people are worried about the possible side effects of treatment. All treatments cause some side effects. But side effects vary from one person to another. Treatments for leukaemia are continuing to improve, which means that more people are surviving with fewer side effects. There are medicines to help control most side effects that happen during or straight after treatment. Many of these effects stop when the treatment ends.

Side effects might be immediate or long term.

Immediate side effects

Immediate side effects happen when you have the treatment or very soon after you finish. The immediate side effects depend on which treatments you have. Some common side effects of acute lymphoblastic leukaemia treatment include:

- low resistance to infection
- anaemia
- risk of bruising and bleeding
- tiredness (fatigue)
- a sore mouth
- taste changes
- changes in your heart muscle
- complete hair loss
- women's periods usually stop and men might stop producing sperm

Late effects

Late effects are medical conditions that develop some years after treatment, for example, heart disease, clouding of the eye lens (cataracts), or not being able to have children (infertility). Because treatments have improved, the treatment that people have now is less likely to cause long term problems than treatment in the past.

Coping with late effects

It can be difficult to cope with problems that develop after treatment. You might feel that it's very unfair to have to cope with side effects as well as the leukaemia and its treatment. Some people find that talking through these issues can help them to cope. It can also help to know about the risk of developing late effects. Keeping as healthy as possible can help to reduce the chance of some problems developing. This includes not smoking, eating a well-balanced diet, keeping a healthy weight and exercising regularly.

Long terms side effects of treatment

The long term side effects of treatment for acute lymphoblastic leukaemia (ALL) and how to cope with them. After some types of leukaemia treatment you might develop long term effects weeks, months or years after the treatment has ended. Different types of treatment cause different problems. And unfortunately doctors can't tell who will get a long term effect and who won't.

Your risk of developing any effect depends on:

- the type of treatment you had
- the treatment dose
- your age when you had treatment

It does not mean having one doesn't mean that you will

develop the others. There are differences between the effects that adults have compared to children. There is less information about adults because acute leukaemia is rarer in adults.

Possible side effects

- Problems with fertility
- Second cancer
- Lung problems
- Clouding of the eye lens (cataract)
- Tiredness (fatigue)
- Low resistance to infection
- Heart problems
- Thyroid problems
- Memory and concentration changes
- Thinning of the bones (osteoporosis)
- Problems specific to children

As well as the possible side effects listed above, there are particular effects in children treated for leukaemia. A transplant in childhood may cause delayed growth due to lower growth hormone levels. Doctors or specialist nurses keep a close eye on children during check-ups to make sure they are growing normally. You might need to see a doctor called an endocrinologist who specialises in hormones.

Children may have puberty later than normal.

Coping with late effects

It can be difficult to cope with problems that develop after treatment. You might feel that it's very unfair to have to cope with side effects as well as the leukaemia and its treatment. Some people find that talking through these issues can help them to cope. It can also help to know about the risk of developing late effects. Ask your specialist doctor or nurse about possible side effects. Keeping as healthy as possible can help to reduce the chance of some problems developing. This includes not smoking, eating a well-balanced diet, keeping a healthy weight and exercising regularly.

www.ingramcontent.com/pod-product-compliance
Lightning Source LLC
Chambersburg PA
CBHW031615210526
45464CB00004B/1589